High Blood Pressure Lowered

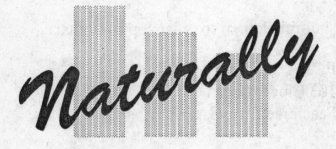

Naturally

U.S. Edition
by the Staff of FC&A

The Natural Way to Help Control Your Blood Pressure, With Your Doctor's Permission

For information, or to order copies, contact:

FC&A Publishing
103 Clover Green
Peachtree City, GA 30269

Publisher: FC&A Publishing
Text: Janice McCall Failes and Frank W. Cawood
Editor: Belinda Kent
Production: Carol Parrott
Cover Design: Deberah Williams
Printed and bound by Banta Company

Second revised printing January 1993

ISBN 0-915099-45-4

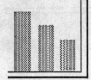

TABLE OF CONTENTS

Pleasant words are like a honeycomb, sweetness to the soul and health to the body.

-PROVERBS 16:24

For I will restore health to you, and your wounds will I heal, says the Lord.

-JEREMIAH 20:17a

WARNING!

High blood pressure is a serious disease. Check with your doctor before discontinuing any medication or trying to treat yourself.

1

INTRODUCTION

High blood pressure, or hypertension, is one of modern society's worst enemies. It is estimated that almost 60 million Americans have some form of this disease. It is a subtle condition, often with no obvious symptoms in its early stages, yet people with high blood pressure are three to five times more vulnerable to heart attacks than those with normal blood pressure. Although it is rarely listed on death certificates as the cause of death, high blood pressure, if left untreated, can lead to many other causes of death. Strokes, heart attacks, kidney failure and blindness are major examples of the devastation of this elusive disease. By reducing blood pressure five or six points (millimeters of mercury) for a few years, the risk of coronary heart disease can be lowered by 14 percent and the risk of stroke by 42 percent, according to a report in *The Lancet* (335:827).

With all these complications, high blood pressure might be the country's leading cause of death. However, many high blood pressure victims are unaware they have the disease. Education about its seriousness and its many known causes is half the battle against the disease.

The purpose of this book is to do just that — to educate. You will learn what high blood pressure is and what it can do to you, the types of drugs used to treat it, and lifestyle changes you can make to control it.

High blood pressure can be lowered without drugs. In one university test, over 85 percent of patients with high blood pressure were able to stop taking their medication, and their blood pressures were lower than when they were taking drugs. The hundreds of people in the study also found that their blood cholesterol levels dropped 26 percent.

You might also be able to cut your risk of developing high blood pressure by making moderate changes in lifestyle, scientists indicate in a report in the *Journal of the American Medical Association* (262,13:1801).

The researchers studied 201 men and women who were slightly overweight, ate salty foods, smoked, downed several alcoholic drinks a day, and rarely exercised. All of them had blood pressure in the "high-normal" range. That means a diastolic (lower number) pressure of from 80 to 99 mm Hg. But, otherwise, they were all healthy.

These prime candidates for high blood pressure agreed to work on better nutrition and to shoot for four goals: lose at least 10 pounds, reduce daily salt intake to less than one-tenth of one ounce, cut back to no more than two alcoholic drinks a day, and exercise for 30 minutes three times per week. Smokers were advised to quit. The researchers encouraged the study participants to stick to a low-fat diet recommended by the American Heart Association.

For five years, the participants — ranging in age from 30 to 44 — kept food diaries, visited their doctors regularly, were given blood and urine tests, and had their blood pressures checked periodically. Three-quarters of them exercised faithfully, mostly walking, jogging and cycling. One out of four met the weight-loss goal, but fewer than two in 10 reduced salt intakes. All said they averaged no more than two drinks a day. They cut their daily calorie intake by an average of 800 calories, a drop of 30 percent. They cut back modestly on saturated fat and cholesterol.

During the same period, physicians kept track of another, similar group that took no special dietary, weight-loss or exercise measures. In other words, just everyday people who continued to eat, drink and do what they pleased.

After five years, the researchers found that the "do-as-you-please" group had double the rate of high blood pressure as the study group. The nutritional approach also helped those in the study group who did develop high blood pressure by delaying its onset for a year or more in most cases. Those who lost the most weight experienced the most benefits, the researchers report. On the negative side, smokers were nearly four times as likely to develop high blood pressure as non-smokers, the report indicates.

One in five people in the "do-as-you-please" group developed high blood pressure during the five-year trial, compared with one in 11 in the nutrition study group. That proved true even though most people in the study group did not reach their original goals.

There is a lot you can do to help your doctor care for you even if you are already taking medication. First, we must emphasize that you should never stop taking your medication on your own. This can cause very serious problems.

Work with your doctor. Let him help you try to become free of the medications and only employ natural methods with his consent. Your doctor will monitor your progress and help you alter your prescriptions safely.

If you have high blood pressure, be sure to carefully consult with your doctor before discontinuing medication or treating the condition yourself.

2

Blood Pressure Defined

What is blood pressure?

Every time your heart beats, it pumps oxygen-rich blood through the arteries to feed every cell in the body with vital nutrients. The "used" blood is then transported through the veins, cleansed in the kidneys and lungs and then back to the heart to begin the cycle again. Blood pressure is the force exerted on the walls of the arteries, veins and capillaries as the heart pumps blood through the body. Without enough pressure, blood would not be able to pick up oxygen from the lungs or force impurities through the kidneys to the bladder. The body must always maintain enough blood pressure for essential functions.

How is blood pressure measured?

Blood pressure is usually taken with an arm-pressure cuff, called a sphygmomanometer (which comes from two Greek words that mean pulse measurement). Blood pressure is taken in two readings: e.g., 120/80. The first number refers to systolic pressure, or the pressure which is produced as the heart contracts to pump blood out into the body. The second number refers to diastolic pressure, or the pressure which remains in the blood vessels as the heart relaxes to allow blood to flow into the pumping chamber (the left ventricle of the heart).

Blood pressure is measured in millimeters of mercury, abbreviated as mm Hg. Mercury is used as a standard because it is much heavier than blood or water (13.6 times heavier), and its rises and falls accurately show the rises and falls in blood pressure. Mercury was first used to measure blood pressure by Jean Leonard-Marie Poiseuille in Paris in 1828, and it continues to be used for blood pressure measurement today.

When someone takes your blood pressure, a tightly fitting cuff is wrapped around your upper arm. Air is pumped into the cuff which stops the flow of blood in your arm. A stethoscope is placed on the arm over the artery. While the cuff is inflated, nothing is heard because the blood flow has been completely cut off. As a valve is turned and the air begins to escape from the cuff, the first pulse sound is heard through the stethoscope. The height of the mercury or the number on the gauge is noted when the first pulse is heard. This is the systolic level. As the air continues to be released from the cuff, the pulse sounds get stronger, then fade. When they fade, another steady sound is heard. This is the sound of the blood flowing through the veins. The number on the gauge at this point is your diastolic pressure.

Electronic or digital gauges have replaced the traditional column of mercury in most new blood pressure measuring devices. Automatic blood pressure monitors, where a cuff is automatically inflated around your arm at regular intervals and the blood pressure noted, are also becoming popular. Automatic monitors, known as ambulatory monitors, can be worn throughout the day and provide accurate readouts for the doctor under different conditions, like working, sleeping and resting blood pressure levels.

The most accurate way of measuring blood pressure is having a catheter inserted into an artery. The catheter's electronic signal is recorded, and the blood pressure is measured. This is sometimes used in people with hardening of the arteries to get more precise readings.

Recording the full range of blood pressure, including the systolic highs and the diastolic resting pressure, may be the next step in diagnosing high blood pressure. A new monitor being developed at the Technion-Israel Institute of Technology in Haifa, Israel, will eliminate the need for the arm cuff and stethoscope. The experimental monitor uses a small wristband that is more comfortable than a cuff, according to its developers. Also, the reading will be taken in just one second, compared to more than a minute needed for present monitoring. Sensors in the new monitor will give doctors a printout of "waves" of blood pressure, providing more information than current techniques.

A similar method, which records the sounds of the blood pulsing through the veins in a continuous wave of blood pressure levels, is now being researched at the Cardiovascular Center of Cornell University Medical College. Rather than having only the high (systolic) and the low (diastolic) readings, the waves will show a continuous reading of all the blood pressure levels on a printed graph.

What blood pressure levels are considered normal?

"Normal" blood pressure readings are based on average blood pressures for different age groups. Generally, blood pressures increase as people get older. Thus a pressure reading, for example, of 139/89 might be considered normal for someone over 50 but too high for a younger person. Regardless of age, blood pressure at or above 140/90 which is sustained for a long period of time is considered high and will damage the body.

If the lower (diastolic) number is between 90 to 104, the high blood pressure is considered mild. Moderate is from 105 to 114, and severe is anything above 115, according to the National Heart, Lung and Blood Institute. Severe high blood pressure, more than 250/115, calls for immediate attention and should be treated as an emergency.

Many people are told they have a "borderline" case of high blood pressure. Usually these people have levels that are at the high end of "normal" or in the "mild" classification (140 to 150 systolic or 90 to 104 diastolic). Most doctors will not prescribe drugs at this stage but will encourage lifestyle changes to lower the blood pressure naturally, before it causes damage to the vital organs.

Both numbers are used to evaluate blood pressure problems, but the diastolic level is still considered the most important. However, a new report shows that a systolic number of 160 or more doubles the risk of stroke or heart attack even if the diastolic number is within the normal range. Usually both numbers will rise if high blood pressure is present, but now if someone has a high reading in either their diastolic or systolic levels, they should be treated for high blood pressure, warns Boston University's Dr. William Kannel.

What is essential hypertension?

Essential hypertension is the most common type, affecting about 90 to 95 percent of high blood pressure victims. The causes are not known, but there may be several factors elevating blood pressure levels, such as a diet high in salt and fat, smoking and family history.

In approximately 5 to 10 percent of cases, high blood pressure can be caused by other diseases, like kidney artery disease, Cushing's disease, brain tumors, narrowing of the aorta (the main artery in the body), or tumors of the adrenal glands. This is called secondary hypertension as it is the result of another disease. The only way to treat this kind of hypertension is for your doctor to treat the disease causing it.

Some people have low blood pressure which can cause unusual tiredness but doesn't damage the body like high blood pressure. People with low blood pressure tend to live longer than average.

What are the symptoms of high blood pressure?

The symptoms of high blood pressure are often silent. It may have no obvious symptoms in its early stages. Often, high blood pressure may be detected only by having the blood pressure taken. Later, as high blood pressure damages the body, many health problems may show up. Symptoms such as depression, ringing in the ears, fainting spells, flushing of the face, headaches, tension, dizziness, nosebleed or blurred vision may be experienced. Since these traits are so general, and most people with normal blood pressure can experience them, the symptoms are not a reliable way to detect high blood pressure.

Forty percent of people with high blood pressure are unaware they have it, according to statistics from the Virginia Department of Health. Twenty percent know but are not participating in therapy. Another 20 percent are receiving treatment, but their blood pressure isn't fully controlled. Only 20 percent of victims are aware they have high blood pressure and have it under control through proper treatment.

You cannot feel that you have high blood pressure — you must have your blood pressure checked regularly.

3

GETTING IT CHECKED

When should blood pressure be checked?

In people with normal blood pressure levels, blood pressure should be taken a minimum of once a year, but twice a year is preferable. People at highest risk, those with parents who have had high blood pressure, blacks and people who are overweight should have it checked at least every six months.

If you have high blood pressure and your doctor recommends diet, losing weight and exercise as the first steps in control, your blood pressure should be monitored at least once every two weeks.

If a prescription drug is prescribed, the doctor may want to monitor your blood pressure twice a week until the effects of the drug are known. If the drug provides a stable blood pressure, it may only need to be checked every few months.

Blacks of all ages and women taking birth control pills should have their blood pressure checked at least twice a year. The first time "the pill" is taken your blood pressure should be monitored every other month for the first year.

Everyone, even children, should be tested. High blood pressure not only can be harmful by itself, but it can also be a symptom of other serious conditions, like heart disease or kidney disease.

Who should take your blood pressure?

Your doctor should be the person to check your blood pressure, but not everyone goes to a doctor regularly. Some sports centers and supermarkets have monitoring machines, or you may want to buy your own device for home use. You can buy a standard sphygmomanometer or an electronic one that is battery operated and usually far easier to use.

For many people on blood pressure medication, monitoring is often required twice a week. If these people can learn to take their blood pressure readings at home, they could save themselves a lot of money, while providing the doctor with more valuable readings.

Should it be taken at home?

In many cases, blood pressure readings are higher in the doctor's office than they are at home. Physicians at the New York Hospital-Cornell University Medical College compared home blood pressure monitoring to levels recorded in the doctor's office. "Home readings were lower and more accurate ... and reflect the overall level of blood pressure more reliably than office readings," the physicians concluded in *Hypertension* (6:574).

Many physicians are now encouraging their patients with high blood pressure to monitor their own levels and record them at home. Patients bring their blood pressure "diary" to each checkup. This way, the doctor can evaluate the blood pressure based on the normal daily blood pressure, rather than on an inflated blood pressure reading taken during a stressful visit to the doctor's office. Higher office readings have been referred to as "white coat hypertension" (*Journal of the American Medical Association* 247:992), because blood pressure sometimes rises when patients feel stressed by a visit to the doctor.

Taking your blood pressure at home can also provide the doctor with more information since more readings can be taken and because home readings are more convenient. A report in the *British Medical Journal* (285:1691) says that home blood pressures are as accurate as clinic readings and, because they are recorded more frequently, they provide more useful information.

James Lynch, director of the Psychophysiological Clinic at the University of Maryland Medical School, urges all patients to take their blood pressure at home, at work and during different stressful situations. All readings should be recorded with any unusual circumstances noted. Lynch finds that knowing their blood pressure levels helps people learn their own reactions to stress and what everyday activities increase their blood pressure.

Home monitoring itself can be a factor in lowering your blood pressure. A study in Seattle showed blood pressure levels lowered by 10 mm Hg or more in 43 percent of people when they monitored their blood pressure at home. The researchers believe that regular monitoring fosters an increased awareness of blood pressure and helps the patient remember that he has a serious problem. He then works harder to make lifestyle changes that will improve his health.

How do you take a blood pressure reading?

Anyone can learn to take blood pressure readings accurately. It is easier to have someone else take your reading, but even people living alone can take their readings at home with the right equipment and a little practice.

All sphygmomanometers will come with instructions, but here are a few tips that you can apply no matter what type you buy:

- Wrap the cuff around your arm so that it is snug, but not uncomfortable.
- Pump enough pressure into the cuff to cut off the blood supply (about 200 to 225 mm on the gauge). It will probably feel like your arm is being squeezed very tightly.
- While taking the measurement, rest your elbow on a table at about heart level.
- Take more than one measurement.

What can cause an inaccurate reading?

Great stress, physical exercise and the time of day can all affect your blood pressure levels. Don't smoke just before your blood pressure is checked because smoking can cause a higher reading. Don't walk up stairs or walk briskly to your doctor's appointment. It is best to be calm and relaxed and in a resting position for about five minutes before your blood pressure is taken.

Your position during a blood pressure reading is very important. If you raise your arm when your blood pressure is taken, the level will often be lower than if you let your arm hang down at your side. If you stand, it will be different than if you are sitting or lying down. The most accurate way to measure blood pressure is to sit down with your arm resting on a table level with your heart.

Most of the time, blood pressure is measured in your right arm. However, blocked arteries or other problems in your arm may cause inaccurate blood pressure readings. The first time your blood pressure is measured, it should be taken in both arms and both readings should be recorded, including the arm that was used. Then, if the readings are similar, the right arm can be used for future monitoring.

If the stethoscope is pressed into the arm with too much force, the diastolic blood pressure reading can be as much as 10 percent too high, reveals the *Western Journal of Medicine* (141:193). The stethoscope needs to be pressed against the artery with firm, but gentle, pressure, the article warns, or you may be needlessly treated for high blood pressure.

Overweight people or people who are very tiny, like children, might need a different cuff than the standard size. A regular cuff is usually between 4 3/4 and 5 inches wide. An overweight person needs a special cuff which is over 6 inches wide, and children need a narrow cuff for accurate readings.

What is false high blood pressure?

Many people diagnosed as having high blood pressure are wrongly diagnosed. Researchers in Canada found that "one of every four people who appeared to have high blood pressure actually did not." Dr. Nicholas Birkett, the study's chief researcher, speculates that those people experienced "white coat hypertension" — nervousness at being in the presence of a physician. This caused their blood pressure to be unusually high during the doctor's visit.

When blood pressure was taken twice more on two separate occasions, the people were found to have normal blood pressure.

Dr. Birkett's finding has been confirmed by investigators at New York Hospital - Cornell University Medical Center (*Journal of the American Medical Association* 259:225). They compared blood pressure measurements obtained by doctors with readings taken by an automatic arm recorder worn during the day. For both hypertensive patients and those with normal blood pressure, the highest blood pressure recorded was the one taken by the doctor. Blood pressure levels taken by a nurse were lower, and the levels recorded on the automatic recorder worn at home were even lower.

Women are most likely to be misdiagnosed as having high blood pressure when their levels are taken by a male doctor, the Cornell study shows. Levels are more accurate when taken by a technician, although the researchers aren't sure why. Dr. Thomas G. Pickering, one of the researchers, suggests that the doctor is seen as more of an authority figure and causes more anxiety than a technician. They conclude that many women, especially younger women, who are classed as having high blood pressure are misdiagnosed. They really have normal levels. Having a woman doctor or technician take the reading can give a more accurate level.

Dr. Lawrence Krakoff, of the Mount Sinai Medical Center, often uses ambulatory monitors which can be worn throughout the day to provide accurate readouts under different conditions, like working, sleeping and resting. Fifty percent of his patients with mild high blood pressure have lower diastolic levels when an ambulatory monitor is used, Dr. Krakoff explains.

Hardening of the arteries in the elderly may also cause high, inaccurate blood pressure readings, according to Dr. Frank H. Messerli, a blood pressure specialist, who was quoted in *The New England Journal of Medicine* (312:1548).

Dr. Messerli discovered that people over 65 with hardened arteries had higher blood pressure when monitored with a blood pressure cuff rather than using a needle inside the arteries.

For an accurate diagnosis of mild high blood pressure, Dr. Birkett recommends taking three or four separate readings over as long as six months. Home blood pressure readings or 24-hour monitoring can help give physicians a better picture of a patient's true blood pressure.

4

WHO GETS IT?

Who gets high blood pressure?

The exact cause of high blood pressure is a mystery in about 90 percent of all cases. We know many of the factors that can lead to high blood pressure, but they might not affect certain people.

For example, someone with a history of high blood pressure in his family who is overweight and smokes might not ever develop high blood pressure. Yet another person with few risk factors may have extremely high blood pressure. Usually though, most people can lower their blood pressure by changing the factors that can be controlled, even if they have other risk factors that they can't control.

Heredity

Children who have one parent with high blood pressure have a greater chance of developing the disease than children with no family history of high blood pressure. When both parents have high blood pressure, the odds are even greater. Check out your parents' and their immediate family's health histories. This does not mean that just because your parents have high blood pressure you will automatically get it — as long as you take care of yourself. If you are at high risk, you should take extra care in your diet, exercise program and lifestyle.

A new genetic screening test might eventually make it possible to identify people at risk for high blood pressure before clinical signs of disease appear, the *Medical World News* reports.

Researchers in California and Michigan have discovered "genetic markers" which signal "increased risk for hypertension and atherosclerosis," the article says.

Dr. Phillipe Frossard, project director at California Biotechnology, has identified 14 markers for hypertension so far, focusing on genes involved with regulating blood pressure. A link between the markers and hypertension is being studied in 70 high blood pressure patients and 30 with normal blood pressure at Cornell University Medical Center.

Frossard believes that genetic testing to predict high blood pressure in people with no symptoms will become routine within the next few years.

Not only will accurate prediction of high blood pressure and atherosclerosis enable physicians to truly "practice preventative medicine," Frossard says, but also the prescribed treatment will be more effective if the doctor knows "what genetic defect is causing the problem."

In separate research, Dr. Brian Robinson at St. George's Hospital in London found that a basic cell defect might be the cause of high blood pressure in about half of the people who develop it. He found that some people with high blood pressure had an abnormal reaction to calcium in their muscle cells *(American Journal of Cardiology).* Robinson hopes to be able to identify who has these cell defects and how their blood pressure can be properly regulated.

Race

Four times as many black Americans develop high blood pressure as white Americans. One of every four blacks has high blood pressure, compared to one of every six Americans overall, the National Heart, Lung and Blood Institute reports. Researchers are not sure what causes the difference, but high blood pressure is usually more severe in blacks, starts earlier and can lead to more severe complications, like premature strokes. High blood pressure and its related diseases are the major cause of death of blacks, according to Max Feinman in *Live Longer.*

One theory that explains racial differences in rates of high blood pressure is that people with ancestors from the tropics where salt is often lacking and fluid loss from perspiration is high are more likely to have a "salt retention gene" than people whose ancestral home was outside the tropics. This "salt retention" gene when it is present in any race causes the body to retain fluids and increase blood pressure.

The following chart shows the estimated rates of prevalence of high blood pressure in blacks and whites, based on the final report of the 1984 Joint National Committee on Detection, Evaluation, and Treatment of High Blood Pressure.

Age	White	Black
65-74	63%	76%
55-64	51%	71%
45-54	39%	62%
35-44	21%	40%
25-34	13%	19%
18-24	9%	10%

Gender

Who do you think of when you picture someone with high blood pressure? Do you think of a middle-age man who is climbing the corporate ladder while supporting a family? Most of us think of men as the main victims of high blood pressure. This may be true in the younger years, but it seems that more women develop high blood pressure later in life. And during life changes like pregnancy and menopause, women are at high risk for developing high blood pressure.

Age

Children and high blood pressure

Dr. Andrew G. Aronfy, a Fellow of the American Academy of Pediatrics (F.A.A.P.), writes:

"Until about 10 to 15 years ago, most pediatricians did not own a blood pressure cuff. In those days, the practice of pediatrics stopped at puberty, and blood pressure measurements were not part of a routine physical examination.

"During the past decade all that has changed. Other doctors started telling pediatricians that many young adults had high blood pressure, and they wondered when it started. When they asked pediatricians for blood pressure readings on their former patients, most pediatricians were embarrassed to confess they had never checked it.

"Secondly, new discoveries about high blood pressure and coronary artery disease revealed that some cases may be strongly influenced by heredity. The tendency toward these diseases can be detected even in early childhood with high blood pressure readings and relatively simple blood tests, such as serum cholesterol and triglycerides. If a hereditary pattern seems to be developing, proper diet, exercise and lifestyle throughout the child's life may help reduce the inherited dangers.

"The most common cause of high blood pressure in children is kidney disease. A high blood pressure reading in a child may be a 'tip-off' that the child needs to be referred to an expert in nephrology to determine if kidney disease is present.

"There are other causes of high blood pressure in children. They are rare, and they are usually related to abnormal hormone production which can be caused by a tumor.

"For all these reasons, all children should have their blood pressure routinely checked from the time they are about 3 years old. If there is a history of high blood pressure or heart disease in the family, children should also have regular appropriate blood tests."

For accurate readings, children usually require a smaller blood pressure cuff. If you are monitoring your family's blood pressure at home, check with your doctor or public health nurse to see if you need a smaller cuff for your children.

If you suffer, or have suffered, from high blood pressure, be careful with your children's intake of salt, according to research published in the journal *Pediatrics*.

The craving for salt is acquired. Do not salt your children's food. Limit the amount of salt you use in food preparation. Limit the children's intake of highly salted foods like canned soups, potato chips, pickles and cured meats. If children do not grow up with salt, they will not crave it, and you will lower their risk of getting high blood pressure in the future.

The elderly and high blood pressure

Some studies indicate that approximately 75 percent of people over 65 have high blood pressure. Authorities on heart and artery disease only recently began to acknowledge the unique aspects of high blood pressure in the older population and, as is often the case with such changes of direction in medicine, there is debate among medical leaders on how to treat the disorder.

"Not so long ago it was fashionable to ignore a little bit of high blood pressure in an elderly person," said Dr. W. McFate Smith, Professor of Epidemiology, University of California School of Public Health, Berkeley. "Limited data establishing the risk of elevated blood pressure in the age group over 65, particularly for women, concern over the presumed greater side effects of drugs in the elderly, and alterations in responsiveness to high blood pressure medications that occur with aging" were some of the rationalizations used, Smith explained.

Many authorities believed that high blood pressure was a physiological consequence of aging which was necessary to carry nutrients and oxygen to vital organs like the brain. Lowering blood pressure could be counterproductive, they argued. A more recent concern was that the quality of life — freedom from possible adverse effects of drug treatment — would be compromised by drug therapy.

In contrast to these views, scientific evidence suggested high blood pressure was a significant risk factor for the elderly, according to Dr. Smith.

"Systolic blood pressure has been shown to be a predictor of coronary heart disease mortality well into the ninth decade, and since considerable life expectancy remains for those who have survived to their senior years, it seems logical to attempt to reduce the risk and preserve independence and life expectancy by controlling blood pressure," he explained. Even a nominal rise in blood pressure in the elderly will lead to a higher occurrence of strokes, according to a study recorded in *Geriatrics* (35:34).

It took some time for researchers to establish the benefits of effective therapy among the elderly. The early literature, which studied stroke survivors and attempted to evaluate the influence of hypertension on stroke recurrence, provided inconsistent and conflicting information on the value of therapy, Dr. Smith noted. However, he pointed out, well-controlled clinical trials published in the last decade without exception show a reduction in the risk of stroke and suggest reduction in death rates.

"Treatment should take into account the combined effects of aging and high blood pressure on the cardio-vascular system and the kidneys," said Dr. Abrams, a researcher in the area of blood pressure and the elderly.

According to Dr. Abrams, the major age-related heart and artery changes are stiffening of the arterial system (hardening of the arteries) which can lead to a progressive rise in systolic blood pressure. This can result in thickening of the muscle in the wall of the left ventricle of the heart, a condition known as left ventricular hypertrophy (enlarged heart), frequently seen in old age.

Diuretics seem to be the most effective drugs in the

treatment of elderly hypertensive patients, according to a study conducted by the Medical Research Council. The study, reported in the *British Medical Journal* (304,6824:405), found that diuretics were more effective than beta blockers at controlling high blood pressure, and they significantly reduced heart problems.

Researchers reviewing this, and other studies done over the past few years, confirmed that diuretics are usually the best choice for older patients, although sometimes combinations are needed.

Diabetics

Occasionally, some diabetics will develop high blood pressure. Because insulin helps the kidneys retain sodium, people who have an excess of insulin might also have an excess of sodium, even if they try to reduce salt in their diet. People who are overweight, eat a lot of sugar, or diabetics who might not have adequate control over their insulin levels should watch their blood pressure levels closely.

5

Is It Serious?

How serious is high blood pressure?

Compared to people with normal blood pressure, people with uncontrolled high blood pressure have:

—seven times as many strokes

—four times as much congestive heart failure

—three times as much coronary heart disease

Heart attacks, the largest single cause of death in the United States, account for 36 percent of all deaths among males ages 35 to 64.

High blood pressure is a major risk factor associated with development of cardiovascular disease. Just as too much air pressure can damage the lining and surface of your car's tires, persistent high blood pressure can damage the interior and exterior of your arteries. It can also damage key organs, such as the brain, heart, kidneys and eyes. High blood pressure can also cause additional strain on the body and cause weak body parts to fail.

Strokes

Strokes are the third leading cause of death in most industrialized populations, according to *The Lancet* (33,8789:342). Strokes account for about 10 to 12 percent of deaths, and of those, 88 percent occur in people over age 65. People with high blood pressure, people with a family or personal history of heart disease or strokes, diabetics, smokers, women taking oral contraceptives and men are also at high risk of having a stroke.

Atrial fibrillation is also a risk factor for stroke and transient ischemic attacks (TIA). TIA is a temporary interference of the blood supply to the brain which doesn't result in brain damage but is sometimes a predictor of stroke. Atrial fibrillation occurs when the top chambers of the heart contract rapidly and irregularly. This condition can be caused by high blood pressure or heart disease and is fairly common in the elderly according to *Drug Therapy* (22,8:85).

Controlling high blood pressure can reduce your risk of stroke, researchers reported in the *Journal of the American Medical Association* (258:214-217). They found that "as control of high blood pressure increased the stroke rates decreased." In the study, "controlled" blood pressure referred to levels below 95 mm Hg diastolic. It did not matter if the blood pressure was controlled through prescription drugs or natural methods as long as it was below 95.

A stroke occurs when blood vessels become blocked and cut off the flow of blood to the brain, or when blood vessels break and allow blood to leak into brain tissue. If the brain is deprived of blood, the brain cells die and cannot be replaced. Permanent damage or death can occur. It may take years for high blood pressure to weaken and damage blood vessels, but a stroke can happen within seconds with no warning. A stroke can last for just a few minutes, or it can last for hours.

If the right part of the brain is damaged by a stroke, the person could be paralyzed on the left side and experience a loss in perception, spacing and memory. If the left part of the brain is damaged, the victim could be paralyzed on the right side and have difficulty with speech and remembering words.

If you are at high risk for stroke, you should learn the early warning signs and be prepared to report them to your doctor immediately. Here are some of the signs of a stroke, as identified by the American Heart Association:

- change in vision, like a flash of blindness or double vision
- difficulty with speech
- unexplained headaches or dizziness
- impaired judgement
- numbness, weakness or tingling sensations
- sudden change in mental abilities
- sudden change in personality
- any symptoms that seem to occur only on one side of the body.

However, you can reduce your risk of having a stroke if you lower high blood pressure, control diabetes, stop smoking, lose weight and begin a healthy low-fat, low-salt diet.

Coronary artery disease

Coronary artery disease kills more people in our society than any other illness. What causes it? "Uncontrolled high blood pressure is the biggest risk factor in coronary artery disease," explains Sandy Sorrentino, Ph.D., author of *Coping With High Blood Pressure.*

Coronary artery disease begins when fatty streaks form in the inner linings of the coronary arteries, the arteries which feed blood to the heart muscle. Autopsies show that fatty streaks can begin in the main artery of the body, the aorta, in infancy. These buildups are frequently found in the smaller coronary arteries by the time children become teenagers.

The fatty streaks may build into atheromas, which are small raised plaques of mushy cholesterol, fat and "foam cells" on the inner walls of the arteries. As the plaques grow, they may start to come together and seriously constrict the flow of blood within the arteries. Scar tissue may begin to grow under the fatty plaque, and this scar tissue may become "hardened" by deposits of calcium. This hardening of the arteries is called atherosclerosis. At this point the arteries have reached an advanced state of disease, and the flow of blood may be severely constricted by hard, chalky plaque, which may not regress or shrink even with the best of care.

High blood pressure speeds the development of atherosclerosis, and the hardened arteries, in turn, increase the blood pressure. Also, high cholesterol levels, smoking and being overweight are all causes of high blood pressure and atherosclerosis.

Atherosclerosis is also a major cause of heart attacks and heart problems. Heart attacks may happen after a piece of an atherosclerotic plaque comes loose and plugs a coronary artery or after a partial blockage from atherosclerosis upsets the rhythm of the heartbeat. During a heart attack, the heart may suddenly stop pumping blood effectively or go into a series of ineffective, twitching contractions called fibrillation. Fibrillation often can be stopped by an electrical shock given through the wall of the chest by an electronic defibrillator. After defibrillation, the heart may recover its normal beat.

The survival of a heart attack victim depends upon the severity of the attack and upon the swiftness of medical attention. Coronary intensive care units in larger hospitals are well-equipped to handle heart attack emergencies.

Knowing the warning signs of a heart attack may save your life, especially if you do not delay in seeking medical help. Some heart attacks are called silent heart attacks because there is no advance warning. However, many heart attacks are not unexpected because the victim has suffered, perhaps for years, from angina pectoris or pain in the chest. If a heart attack is not occurring, angina usually will go away after a few minutes of rest or after the administration of doctor-prescribed nitroglycerin, which is taken to dilate or expand the coronary arteries. Since people with high blood pressure are at increased risk for having a heart attack, be sure you know the symptoms:

- heavy pressure or a choking or squeezing sensation in the center of the chest
- chest pain which may radiate down one or both arms, across the back or up the neck
- shortness of breath
- an unexplained sensation or feeling of fear
- perspiration
- nausea
- dizziness or lightheadedness
- weakness or a fainting sensation
- angina pain that lasts for more than a few minutes or that doesn't go away upon administration of nitroglycerin and rest

All of these symptoms need not be present to indicate that a heart attack is taking place.

Heart failure

About 75 percent of high blood pressure victims develop heart failure (the heart can no longer pump blood efficiently), and only 50 percent of patients survive five years after heart failure is detected.

Hypertension is the leading cause of left ventricular hypertrophy which is a major risk factor for heart failure, as well as irregular heartbeat, ischemic heart disease (insufficient blood supply to the heart due to a blockage in the circulation), and sudden death.

Left ventricular hypertrophy is more prevalent in patients with blood pressures of 160/95 mm Hg or higher, according to a report in *The New England Journal of Medicine* (327,14:998).

The risks also increase with age. In the Framingham Heart Study 3 to 7 percent of adults under 50 years of age were found to have left ventricular hypertrophy. That figure went up to 12 to 40 percent in the over-50 population.

Black people with high blood pressure had twice the prevalence of left ventricular hypertrophy as white people with similar blood pressures. "Hypertension was the most common precursor of coronary heart failure in the Framingham Study," say researchers.

The *NEJM* report raises the question of whether reversal of left ventricular hypertrophy would increase survival rates for people with heart problems. The scientists suggest that we should prevent left ventricular hypertrophy from developing, which means controlling blood pressure levels before any damage is done.

A new study reported in the *Archives of Internal Medicine* (152,9:1855) suggests that higher nighttime blood pressure levels are linked to increased organ damage, particularly left ventricular hypertrophy. Researchers studied 728 people using ambulatory monitors, and also found that people with variable daytime blood pressure levels had more cardiovascular problems.

High blood pressure can also cause congestive heart failure. The weakened heart cannot pump blood efficiently so blood flow is restricted, more blood accumulates in the heart and a back-pressure builds up. Fluid builds up in the body's tissues (known as edema), particularly the lower body, and the ankles will probably swell. A person with congestive heart failure will probably experience weakness, breathlessness and abdominal pain. Congestive heart failure affects 3 to 5 percent of people over 65 reports *The Lancet* (339,87:278).

Kidney problems

Uremia, a condition in which the blood becomes toxic due to the kidneys' inability to remove waste products, can be caused by uncontrolled high blood pressure. The high blood pressure causes the arteries to become tighter and more narrow, which eventually reduces the blood pressure to the kidneys. The malfunctioning kidney responds by trying to increase the blood pressure, creating more problems.

Once the kidneys begin to function below normal, waste products like salt are not properly excreted. With salt and other normally excreted products remaining in the kidney, it continues to malfunction. When the kidneys become damaged, they cannot be repaired. Kidney dialysis or a transplant can be used to solve the problem, but sudden death due to kidney failure could also occur.

Controlling blood pressure can prevent irreparable

damage to your kidneys.

Brain damage

Serious swelling of the brain can occur with uncontrolled high blood pressure. A person with a long history of uncontrolled high blood pressure or someone who experiences unusually high blood pressure is at greatest risk. Brain damage or death could occur if the swelling is not treated immediately.

Loss of vision

Just like blood vessels in the brain and throughout the body, high blood pressure also forces the small blood vessels in the eye to narrow. The capillaries in the eyes may begin to deteriorate due to lack of blood and a loss of vision, sometimes called "tunnel vision," or blindness can result.

The relationship between uncontrolled high blood pressure and loss of vision has been verified. Doctors are now aware of the importance of regular eye checkups as well as the monitoring of blood pressure levels when treating people with elevated blood pressure.

Higher death rates in cancer patients

High blood pressure has been associated with higher death rates in cancer patients (*Journal of the National Cancer Institute* 77:1,63). The higher the blood pressure, the more likely the patient was to die from the cancer, the researchers discovered.

The risk factors that might cause high blood pressure, such as a high-fat, high-salt diet or smoking, can also contribute to cancer.

Other risk factors

Although we usually don't know the cause of hypertension, there are other coronary risk factors present in most patients that may contribute to higher blood pressure levels. The following table lists some of the risk factors for coronary diseases and the percentage of hypertensive people who have them.

Sedentary lifestyle	50%
Hyperinsulinemia (an excessive amount of insulin in the blood)	50%
Obesity	40%
Hypercholesterolemia (cholesterol levels greater than 240 mg/dl)	40%
Smoking	35%
Low HDL level (the good cholesterol - less than 40 mg/dl)	25%
Diabetes	15%

Source: *Postgraduate Medicine* (91,8:225-226)

6

CHANGING YOUR DIET

You are what you eat

The next few chapters will focus on the foods we eat and how they affect blood pressure. The dietary guidelines we recommend are much like those used by the Pritikin Longevity Centers. Not long ago, a research team from Loma Linda University studied the results of the Pritikin program, which also included moderate daily exercise such as walking.

Overweight patients lost an average of ten pounds or more. Eighty-five percent of the patients who were taking high blood pressure drugs were able to stop taking these drugs with their doctors' permission because their blood pressures had dropped to acceptable levels.

Cholesterol levels dropped 26 percent. Many people who had been taking drugs to control their blood cholesterol were able to stop taking medicine. The level of other blood fats also dropped nearly 26 percent. Forty percent of the patients who were diabetics were able, under medical supervision, to stop taking insulin. The patients became more mentally alert and performed better on tests of mental ability. Many patients lost their tiredness and required much less sleep.

This type of diet works against high blood pressure in three ways:

- It is low in calories so people can lose weight
- It is low in sodium to help sodium-sensitive people
- It is low in cholesterol to help limit damage to the heart and arteries caused by high blood pressure

Before changing your eating habits

Evaluate your present eating habits. Note how many high-sodium, high-calorie and high-cholesterol foods you eat on a daily basis. Look for ways to improve your diet and make a commitment to yourself that you will try to improve your health through your diet.

Consider the effects dietary changes might have on your body. Also, consider the effects a drastic change in eating habits might have on your mind and emotions.

First, don't overdose on fiber. Your body has had years to adjust to the lack of fiber in the typical American diet, and it may take a few days or weeks to become adjusted to higher levels of fiber.

If you have a problem with too frequent elimination or flatulence, cut back a little on high-fiber foods, like bran muffins and bran bread. Substitute foods which contain adequate but lighter fiber, like oatmeal, brown rice or bread made with half whole wheat flour and half unbleached white flour. Each person is unique, so you may have to experiment to find out how much fiber is right for you.

Secondly, if a total change in eating habits is too hard,

gradually change your habits by substituting whole grain cereals for bacon or sausage at breakfast, making sandwiches with whole wheat bread, or pulling the fat-laden skin off of chicken. Many people can move in little steps toward a much more healthy diet.

Your approach to eating the foods that are best for your health needs to be continued throughout your life. By slowly making changes, you might be able to live with them for a longer time. Sometimes, drastic changes in diet are too difficult, and the person completely reverts back to his old eating habits.

Learning what foods are beneficial and what foods should be avoided is the first step. If you are only able to follow the following dietary recommendations in half of the foods you eat, you will still receive a substantial benefit. The more the recommendations are followed, the greater the benefits will be. Even one step in the right direction will be helpful in improving your total health.

At home or in a restaurant, try to eat foods that are lightly cooked: broiled, steamed, roasted or baked in their own juices. Raw fruits and vegetables are also good choices.

Drink about six to eight glasses of water each day. Water is necessary for regular bowel movements, to help flush out sodium, to help prevent kidney stones, to protect us from disease and to prevent dehydration. Drinking "hard" certified pure spring water is recommended. Also, older people need to be especially careful to drink enough water each day, because many elderly people lose their sense of thirst, reports a study in *The New England Journal of Medicine*. Since they may not feel thirsty or uncomfortable, older people can become dehydrated.

Snacking during the day might be better for your heart than eating three square meals a day, Canadian researchers report in *The New England Journal of Medicine* (321,14:929).

But that doesn't mean you can eat just potato chips and ice cream — or simply snack between meals.

To get the benefits, you must eat small, nutritious meals throughout the day, researchers say, and your calorie count must not increase.

Researchers believe snacking works by controlling the production of certain chemicals in the body.

Insulin, a hormone released by the pancreas, helps the body produce cholesterol. How much insulin the pancreas releases into the bloodstream depends on the size of the meals you eat.

Snackers may have lower cholesterol levels because they eat smaller amounts of food, and the pancreas produces less insulin in response.

Less insulin usually means less cholesterol.

Eating more meals throughout the day and adding more fiber to your diet might be keys to keeping your cholesterol levels under control.

During the study, seven men ages 31 to 51 ate three

meals a day for two weeks or 17 snacks a day for two weeks and then switched to the other diet.

The snackers' insulin levels dropped by 28 percent during the study.

Their total cholesterol levels were 8.5 percent lower than men eating three meals a day.

Based on the results of this study, researchers believe that nutritious nibbling throughout the day might help you lower cholesterol levels and fight heart disease.

Foods that are good for you

As a general guide, here is a list of foods that are good for you because they are low in salt, fat and cholesterol.

lean veal   whole wheat noodles
skim milk   lean beef
yogurt (low fat)   olive oil
skim milk cheeses   onions
peppers   vinegar
dried beans   dried rice
dried peas   dried barley
chicken (with skin removed)
fish (packed in water)
baked potatoes (with little or no butter or margarine)
homemade whole-grain yeast bread (made without salt or baking powder)
natural cereals (without salt added)
beverages which don't contain fat or caffeine
fresh fruits and vegetables

cottage cheese (low-fat or dry-curd varieties)

Foods to avoid

Here are some foods and preparations to avoid as you seek to lower your blood pressure naturally.

canned or dried soup	bacon
pickles or olives	cheese
potato chips or pretzels	salted nuts
french fries	most crackers
canned vegetables	sauerkraut
canned meats	liver
smoked meat or fish	shrimp
luncheon meat	lobster
salt-cured ham	herring
pork	sardines
sausage	caviar
pepperoni	anchovies
hot dogs	flavored gelatin
instant cocoa mixes	pizza
most processed food	chocolate milk
"fast food"	ice cream
most frozen dinners	milk shakes
beer	baking powder
tomato sauce and ketchup	baking soda
most sauces	garlic salt
gravy	onion salt
boullion	celery salt
salad dressings	mustard
cake mixes	relish

pancake mixes
muffin mixes
pudding mixes
biscuit mixes
cornbread mixes
peanut butter
MSG (monosodium glutamate)
foods containing sodium bicarbonate
foods containing disodium phosphate
salted butter or salted margarine

horseradish
chili sauce
Worcestershire sauce
soy sauce
many laxatives
meat tenderizer

also ok/with Blood type = beef, buffalo
heart, lamb, liver, mutton,
veal & venison

also avoid = pork, catfish, caviar, lox
octopus

less breads & muffins - only Essene &
Ezekiel Breads ok

7

VITAMINS AND MINERALS

Salt: good and bad news

You may be preparing yourself to hear that one more flavor you love — salt — is bad for your health. Is there nothing you can enjoy eating anymore?

Salt itself isn't bad for your health. You may know that in the Bible Jesus says, "Ye are the salt of the earth," indicating that even thousands of years ago salt was a valuable commodity for preserving food and stimulating taste buds. The word from which we get our word "salary" comes from the Latin word "sal," meaning salt. Roman soldiers were sometimes said to be "worth their salt" because they were often paid in salt rather than actual money.

Why, then, all the fuss about removing salt from our diets? Why is it so bad all of a sudden? Is this a passing medical "fad"?

Unfortunately, the answer is "no." This is not a passing problem. What has happened is that we have simply "overdosed" on a good thing to the point that it has become a bad thing.

A low-sodium diet is one of the basic, natural ways to lower high blood pressure, but many people are hesitant because they think that a salt-free diet is bland. However, researchers at the University of Minnesota discovered that your desire for salt and your taste change when you start a low-salt diet.

"The study was initiated because many participants in earlier studies reported that once they were on a low-sodium diet, many foods that had been acceptable were now 'too salty' or even unpleasant," Dr. Richard Grimm recently announced.

Participants on a low-salt diet compared salted crackers at regular intervals. "The highest-sodium-content crackers were rated more salty and less pleasant," Grimm said.

"The level of sodium preferred also decreased ... these changes in taste occurred early and were evident by the sixth-week visit."

"In questionnaires, men on low-sodium diets reported they were more sensitive to the taste of salt, found many high-salt foods to be unpleasant, and stated that the diet was easier to follow the longer they stayed on it," Grimm explained.

As people reduce the amount of salt in their diets, they experience new flavor sensations that were masked by the large amounts of salt they ate. The true flavor of vegetables can be hidden by cooking with too much salt. In this sense, excessive salt can be a taste destroyer rather than a flavor enhancer.

One scientific study on salt consumption deals with twins. One twin was put on a low-salt diet. The other twin continued to consume a diet high in salt. After a few weeks, the twin on the low-salt diet learned to consume less salt and preferred to eat less salt. The other twin was still in the habit of consuming more salt and continued to prefer the high-salt diet.

Salt is made up of 40 percent sodium and 60 percent chloride. It is essential to life, and it is an important mineral in the body. Without it we would die. Salt maintains fluid levels between the cells and the blood system and acts as an electrolyte to help chemical and electrical reactions in the body.

However, our bodies are equipped to handle only so much salt. Dr. Cleaves M. Bennett, author of *Control Your High Blood Pressure Without Drugs*, says, "The quantities of salt we actually eat are a great burden on our systems. It's so destructive. As we eat more salt than the kidneys can readily excrete, over a long period of time, many years, salt builds up in the body .... The body's way to get rid of more of that salt ... is to push it out through the kidneys by raising the blood pressure."

The average person eats five to 10 grams of sodium, or one-third to one-fifth of one ounce of salt per day. This is much more salt than is needed for bodily functions. Recent studies indicate that some people need as little as one-fifth of one gram (200 milligrams). A healthy amount for most people is from 500 milligrams (mg) up to no more than 1,000 mg of salt per day. However, there are exceptions. Hard labor, profuse sweating, pregnancy and breast-feeding might increase the need for salt up to two grams per day.

Most people will question whether they really consume one-third to one-fifth of an ounce of salt per day, but the processed foods that we all eat are usually filled with salt and can account for up to 75 percent of salt intake. Any food that comes in a can, a frozen package or a box is likely to have salt added as a preservative or flavor enhancer.

Table salt and salty products can be easy to avoid, but it is this "hidden salt" that often has consumers stumped. The Food and Drug Administration (FDA) requires soft-drink manufacturers to list the sodium content of their drinks on the bottles or cans. Many products list their nutritional information, but be wary of their advertising and labeling. The higher up on the ingredients list salt appears, the higher the content. Check labels very carefully. A slice of bread may contain over 200 mg of salt, a bowl of cornflakes over 300 mg, a bowl of canned soup over 1,000 mg, a chicken dinner from a fast food restaurant over 2,000 mg and a large dill pickle over 1,000 mg.

Studies of different nations around the world show that high blood pressure is a problem only in societies where people eat a lot of salt. Although it is mainly sodium we worry about when we think of blood pressure, chloride is also a factor because it is needed for the reabsorption of sodium. (For this reason, when choosing a salt substitute, don't use one that is made only of potassium chloride.)

High blood pressure rates are in direct proportion to the amount of salt consumed. The more salt that a particular society consumes, the greater the number of cases of severe high blood pressure. It is significant that the Greenland Eskimos and the Amazon Indians, who eat very little salt, have very little high blood pressure. But in the north of Japan, high blood pressure is common among the people whose diet contains large amounts of salt. Of course, in such societies other factors may also be at work, but the strong relationship between salt consumption and high blood pressure should not be underestimated.

If you are concerned about giving up flavor in your cooking, a little creativity can help add "spice" to your food while lowering the salt content. You do not have to sacrifice flavor when you cut down on sodium if you follow these suggestions:

- Remove the salt shaker from your table.
- Never use salt in cooking, or reduce your use of salt in recipes by at least one half.
- Use lemon juice on food instead of salt.
- Don't use onion or garlic salt as spices because they are just "flavored" salt. Use real onion or garlic for more flavor without the salt.
- When baking cakes, cookies, pies and puddings, use extracts instead of salt and reduce the sugar.
- Avoid store-bought mixes for biscuits, cakes, pancakes, muffins, cornbread, etc. If you prepare your own, you can control your ingredients.
- Read all labels to determine the sodium content and buy low-sodium products whenever possible. Avoid any additives that contain the word sodium, like sodium chloride, sodium bicarbonate, sodium benzoate, monosodium glutamate (MSG) or others that

contain sodium, like baking soda, baking powder and brine.

- Learn about the many natural herbs, spices, and fruit peels that are available. You may decide to grow your own or experiment with store-bought herbs.
- Use one of several salt-free mixtures of herbs and spices that are available for seasonings.
- Enjoy Mexican, Cajun and Tex-Mex foods. The strong spices give flavor without adding salt. Beware of oriental food — it can be high in MSG which is high in sodium.
- To spice chicken dishes, add fruits such as mandarin oranges or pineapples.
- Marinate chicken, fish, beef or poultry in orange juice or lemon juice. Add a homemade mustard or honey glaze.
- Marinate meat in wine or add wine to sauces or soups. If you thoroughly cook the dish, the alcohol will evaporate, but the flavor will be enhanced.
- Use fresh vegetables whenever possible. However, if you must use canned vegetables, wash them in cool water before using. Rinsing will help remove some of the salt added when processing.
- Just a little green pepper, parsley, paprika or red pepper can add a lot of flavor to a meal.
- Be sure to keep the meals attractive and include a variety of colors and textures. Most people are more tempted to add salt when the meal appears bland.

- Drink water with your meals and avoid soft drinks.
  Soft drinks are high in sugar which dulls your taste
  buds and makes it more difficult to give up salt. Also,
  many carbonated drinks are high in sodium. Even
  some sugar-free soft drinks contain sodium as sodium saccharin, an artificial sweetener.

A test to show how much salt you are really consuming
is available and may help some people monitor or reduce
their sodium intake, reports a study in *Archives of Internal
Medicine* (144:1963-5). Thirty percent of people in the study
had lower salt intake when they were using a chloride titrator
strip at home. If you are not sure of your current salt intake
or if you want to monitor your diet, check with your doctor
about the titrator strip test.

Many scientific studies show that reducing salt intake will
lower blood pressure in most people by a significant amount.
Getting salt intake down into the range of 500 mg of salt per
day helps the most. Reducing salt intake lowers blood
pressure dramatically in some people because they have an
inherited tendency to hold on to salt or sodium. Thus, the
benefits of reduced salt consumption are greatest for some of
the people who need the benefits the most.

Certain people seem to be "salt sensitive," and others are
not as affected by salt, according to studies by Dr. L.K. Dahl
in *Circulation Research* (40:1131-4). He found that some
animals will develop high blood pressure, no matter how
much salt they ingest. However, some people can consume
large quantities of salt and never develop high blood pres-

sure. Since there are no tests to show who is salt retentive and who is not (although some are being developed), health professionals recommend that everyone reduce their salt intake as part of their high blood pressure treatment.

Protective potassium

We know that excess sodium can elevate blood pressure levels. But just as important is our intake of potassium and the ratio of potassium to sodium in our bodies. Unfortunately, societies which have high levels of salt consumption also have low levels of potassium consumption and vice versa.

A recent study at Duke University showed a significant drop in blood pressure in just two months when participants were given potassium, reports Hypertension (9:571-5).

The *British Medical Journal* (301,6751:521-523) reports on an Indian study that also found potassium supplements significantly reduced blood pressure. The researchers also suggest that potassium may lower serum cholesterol, and decrease the risk of stroke. Other researchers agree. *Medical World News* (30,11:30) reports that several separate studies have demonstrated that increasing potassium in the diet can dramatically lower your risk of death from stroke. According to the report, people who ate the most fruits and vegetables had 25 to 40 percent fewer fatal strokes than groups with lower potassium intakes, and women seem to benefit more from a high-potassium diet than men.

Another study reported in *Modern Medicine* (57,11:103-104) confirms the importance of potassium as a blood pressure reducer. As part of the study at the Temple University School of Medicine, 10 men were put on either low-potassium or normal-potassium diets, then given a saline infusion. The blood pressure levels of the men on low-potassium diets were raised significantly while on the diet and were further raised after the saline infusion. The men on the normal-potassium diets did not seem to be affected at all.

Since this and other research indicates that supplemental potassium in the diet helps to lower blood pressure, eat more foods like bananas and citrus fruits, especially grapefruit, which are relatively high in potassium. Potassium is also found in foods like cantaloupe, potatoes, beans, peas, raisins, pineapple juice, tomatoes, pears, apple juice, peaches, apples, meat, milk and nuts. If you try to eat a diet that includes more natural foods, rather than canned or processed foods, you will automatically raise your potassium intake and lower your sodium intake.

People taking some diuretic drugs that reduce natural potassium might also receive a prescription for a potassium supplement.

Most adults need 1,000 to 5,000 mg of potassium daily, depending on salt intake. Potassium supplements should not be used by people who have kidney disease or who are taking a prescription diuretic that is potassium-sparing, because excessive potassium can be harmful or even fatal. Large doses of potassium should be avoided unless prescribed by a doctor because high levels of potassium might cause heart attacks.

Additional calcium

Insufficient calcium can result in higher blood pressure levels. Calcium works on every cell in the body. If there is a deficiency, it can cause these cells to constrict, increasing peripheral resistance (resistance of blood flow through the arteries and veins) and raising blood pressure. One study indicates that people with high blood pressure consume 20 to 25 percent less calcium than people who don't have high blood pressure. Signs of extremely low levels of calcium in the diet are muscle cramps and numbness in the limbs.

Dr. Lawrence Resnick at the New York Hospital-Cornell Medical Center has found a link between people who are salt retentive and calcium supplementation. The more salt seems to affect someone's blood pressure, the more calcium supplements seem to improve their blood pressure, Resnick reports in the *Journal of Hypertension* (4:5182-5). Also, excess sodium seems to make the body excrete calcium, doubling the problem.

Blood pressure dropped a "modest but significant" amount when men with normal blood pressure levels took 1,500 mg of calcium daily, according to research by Roseann Lyle, Ph.D., a professor at Purdue University, reports the *Journal of the American Medical Association* (257:1772-6). Another study, by researchers from Johns Hopkins University School of Medicine, confirmed that the "degree to which blood pressure falls depends on the amount of calcium taken." Although blood pressure usually rises in the last trimester of pregnancy, blood pressure levels remained constant in women who received 1,500 mg of calcium per day *(Obstetrics and Gynecology)*.

The risk of high blood pressure can be reduced by 22 percent in women who take 800 mg of calcium per day, reports a study from Harvard Medical School. Blood pressure in women taking 800 mg per day was compared to women taking just 400 mg per day.

There are other obvious reasons, such as bone density, for getting an adequate supply of calcium. It's no secret that calcium promotes strong teeth and bones — but not just when you're young.

Dr. Robert P. Heany, of Creighton University, notes the importance of calcium in two major stages of life. It helps develop bone mass during the first 30 years of life, and then maintains bone mass during the remaining years of life.

However, as you get older, your body doesn't use calcium as efficiently as when you were young.

That's why you might need more calcium as you age, some researchers suggest.

Menopausal women might need even more calcium because their estrogen loss puts them at greater risk of developing osteoporosis.

For pregnant women, extra calcium might help prevent preeclampsia. This condition results in excessive fluid retention in the mother's body, which can harm the unborn child if not treated.

The Recommended Dietary Allowance (RDA) of calcium is 800 mg per day (1200 mg for pregnant women and nursing mothers), and some experts think it should be more. Most women are not getting enough calcium in their diets. Nutritionists recommend either changing the diet by increasing low-fat dairy products, like skim milk, cottage cheese and yogurt, or taking daily calcium supplements.

Since taking calcium supplements or increasing the amount of calcium in the diet has few harmful side effects, extra calcium could be part of a blood pressure reducing therapy. Dairy products; salmon; sardines; and leafy, green vegetables are the best natural sources of calcium.

Calcium supplementation should be avoided by people who have calcium oxalate kidney stones or by those with high blood levels of calcium which might make them more inclined to develop kidney stones. Excessive amounts of calcium and vitamin D may make it difficult for the body to eliminate extra calcium, which can cause problems. Excessive vitamin D can be dangerous and can cause high blood pressure by promoting the formation of deposits in the arteries. The RDA of vitamin D is 200 I.U. (International Units) per day.

Even if you start taking supplemental calcium, do not stop taking blood pressure medication except on your doctor's advice.

Supplementing magnesium

It is estimated that eight out of every 10 people have a significant deficiency in the mineral, magnesium. As an average person, you probably consume only about 40 percent of the daily amount of magnesium you need. Therefore, you may be subjecting yourself to higher risks of high blood pressure, diabetes, pregnancy problems in women and cardiovascular disease, including abnormal heart rhythms, according to *Science News* (133:356).

Other studies link magnesium deficiency with increased cancer risks, especially cancer of the esophagus (*Maximum Immunity*). Recent research showed abnormally low levels of magnesium in the heart muscles of victims who died from sudden heart attacks, indicating that magnesium plays a previously unsuspected role in preventing or lessening the effects of heart disease (*Popular Nutritional Practices*).

The further good news about this "miracle" mineral is that recent studies involving humans and animals have demonstrated that magnesium-spiked diets decreased the bad effects of pulmonary (lung) high blood pressure, lowered blood cholesterol levels by as much as 33 percent, dramatically reduced migraines and high blood pressure associated with pregnancies, and even prevented the formation of high blood pressure in rats that had been specially treated to make their blood pressures rise.

In another study, researchers found that intravenous solutions of magnesium given to victims immediately after severe heart attacks cut their post-heart attack death rate in half in the critical four weeks following the attacks, when compared to victims who received only IVs without the added magnesium.

The studies strongly suggest that all of us need to take another look at this little-known mineral. While it's been heralded in recent years as an anti-stress mineral, it may be much more important than we realized for maintaining cardiovascular health and for preventing other serious problems, including cancer and high blood pressure.

Most people don't get even half as much magnesium as they need daily, according to studies presented at the 22nd annual Conference on Trace Substances in Environmental Health and reported in *Science News*. "Many people face serious consequences — including death — from preventable magnesium deficiency ..., and contributing to the problem is that this deficiency 'is likely to be silent until it is severe'," according to Mildred S. Seelig, executive director of the American College of Nutrition.

The studies show that higher levels of dietary magnesium not only prevent development of several serious health problems, but also play a definite role in fighting the bad effects of high blood pressure and fat-rich diets.

For example, in animal tests, results showed that high blood pressure caused by too much salt in the diet was actually prevented by adding magnesium to the drinking water at four to eight times the recommended dietary allowance. In another test, rats getting increased magnesium showed few of the ill effects of deliberately caused high blood pressure, while rats without the added mineral had much higher blood pressure, doubled their heart sizes, and suffered three to seven-fold thickening of artery walls, the report said.

In still another test, this time with rabbits on "normal" cholesterol diets, the researchers showed that increasing magnesium levels to about five times recommended dietary allowances resulted in 30 to 40 percent reductions in blood levels of cholesterol and other blood fats when compared to low-magnesium diets. Equally significant, rabbits on high-cholesterol diets got megadoses of magnesium and cut their blood-fat levels by more than half, the study showed.

Migraine headaches and high blood pressure, both problems for many pregnant women, are directly linked to inadequate magnesium levels, according to an East Tennessee State University researcher in a report to the same conference. Low magnesium levels might also contribute to stillbirths, miscarriages, and low-birthweight babies, studies with both humans and animals showed. Magnesium supplements greatly reduced such problems, the report said.

While experts believe more than eight of every 10 people don't get enough magnesium, the highest risk persons are alcoholics and those taking "water pills" (diuretics), digitalis and other heart drugs, and some antibiotics and anti-cancer drugs, according to Seelig. These substances "bind" with magnesium, prevent its absorption into the body, and speed it through the body without letting it have its good effects. Such persons need to check with their doctors about getting a special higher daily supplement of magnesium, the studies suggested.

According to a study reported in *Hypertension* (19,2:175-182), there is evidence to support the theory that magnesium also helps prevent alcohol-induced high blood pressure. Rats given ethanol and magnesium supplements had significantly lower blood pressure levels than rats given ethanol alone.

Soda fans may also cut down their magnesium absorption to harmful levels because of the "binding" effect of the phosphates they contain. For example, a regular 12-ounce soda may bind up to 30 mg of magnesium and flush it out of the body before it can do its good work.

The RDA of magnesium is 350 mg for males over 18 and 280 mg for females. The RDA for pregnant women and lactating (milk-producing) mothers is even higher — up to 355 mg. Three or four sodas per day could cause significant deficiencies in magnesium absorption, even in those few people who take enough of the mineral every day.

Good dietary sources of magnesium are leafy, dark-green vegetables; whole-grain cereals; figs; lemons; grapefruit; corn; almonds and other nuts; seeds; apples; and seafood. People living in "hard water" areas often get lots of magnesium, and, incidentally, they have low rates of heart attacks and lower blood pressure. But people living where drinking water is soft have severe deficiencies.

However, experts say it's hard to get enough of the mineral just by eating the right foods. They suggest that everyone consider taking a daily supplement in tablet form. One researcher said magnesium would be the one supplement he would recommend for everyone.

You should take magnesium with calcium, several studies said. Dolomite is a good, inexpensive supplement that contains both minerals. Take between meals because magnesium neutralizes stomach acid (remember milk of magnesia?) and acts like an antacid.

Few studies show any harmful effects of higher-than-RDA doses of magnesium. Experts suggest no more than 3,000 mg per day for patients who have kidney problems. One study suggested huge doses of magnesium could be linked to excessively low blood pressure and depressed breathing in a few cases. Any long-term use of magnesium in large doses should, of course, be done only with your doctor's knowledge and permission.

The case for magnesium

Magnesium has been shown in studies to help:
- Prevent formation of salt-induced high blood pressure
- Cut blood cholesterol levels
- Stop migraines in pregnant women
- Cut death rates in half for post-heart-attack patients
- Prevent the formation of several forms of cancer
- Increase oxygen use by muscles, leading to better fitness
- Regulate the body's blood sugar metabolism, raising energy levels
- Fight depression and act with calcium as a natural

tranquilizer
- Help prevent heart attacks
- Aid in stopping calcium deposits, kidney stones and gallstones
- Keep teeth healthier

Vitamin C

Vitamin C might play a bigger role in regulating blood pressure than we once thought.

Researchers have discovered that vitamin C might prevent healthy people from developing high blood pressure and might even help lower slightly elevated blood pressure readings to normal levels, according to a report in *Science News* (137,19:292).

Checking 67 healthy men and women ages 20 to 69, researchers at the Medical College of Georgia found that participants with high levels of vitamin C in the blood averaged a blood pressure reading of 104/65.

Others with one-fifth those blood levels of vitamin C — but still within acceptable, healthy levels — averaged blood pressure readings of 111/73, the report says. The "normal" blood pressure reading usually is considered 120/80.

Researchers suggest that the vitamin somehow pushes blood pressure down, keeping levels at or below "normal."

That provides a cushion against blood pressure rising beyond healthy levels.

Even people with established high blood pressure may benefit from more vitamin C, suggest researchers at Tufts

University.

They checked 241 elderly Chinese-Americans and found the same result: the lower the blood levels of vitamin C, the higher the blood pressure.

You can get vitamin C naturally by eating citrus fruits and dark-green vegetables like broccoli. The current RDA for vitamin C is 60 mg, although many people think that number should be higher. If you choose to take a vitamin supplement, be careful not to take over one gram a day, as this can cause kidney stones, gout and diarrhea.

Increasing choline

Choline (a near-vitamin) supplements are reported to help control blood pressure. In a clinical study, one-third of a group of patients with high blood pressure had their blood pressure return to normal after receiving choline supplements. When the supplements were discontinued, their blood pressure rose once again. However, additional studies are needed to confirm that choline alone was responsible.

Lecithin, soybeans, eggs, fish, liver and wheat germ are rich, natural sources of choline. Green vegetables, peanuts, brewer's yeast and sunflower seeds are also good sources.

Niacin

When niacin (vitamin B3) is taken in high dosages, it has been shown to reduce the amount of cholesterol in the blood (*Journal of the American Medical Association*). In a study of heart attack victims, it was found that people who took high doses of niacin had an 11 percent lower death rate than those who did not.

Niacin must be administered in high doses to be effective against heart disease and cholesterol. But, because of the significant side effects of large doses of niacin, it should be taken only under a doctor's supervision. Some people, such as those with high blood pressure, diabetes, gout or ulcers, should not take niacin at all. The niacinamide form of the vitamin should not be used because it does not lower blood fats by a significant amount. Food sources for niacin include yeast, fish, poultry, liver, meat, whole-grain products (except corn which contains an inactive form of niacin), peanuts, potatoes, beans and mushrooms.

8

ARE ALL FATS BAD?

Diets high in fat

Most Americans consume about 40 percent of their total calories from fat. High-fat diets along with other factors can cause hardening of the arteries which leads to higher and higher blood pressure over the years. Low-fat diets are associated with low blood pressure. Cutting fat intake levels in half can have a dramatic effect in reducing many cases of high blood pressure. A recent study by the U.S. Department of Agriculture found that eating less saturated fat could bring blood pressure down even in the absence of taking other beneficial measures.

Educating yourself to identify and avoid high-fat foods and increasing your fiber intake are two of the most important steps you can take in changing to a healthier diet.

It is important to learn that all fats are not the same.

Saturated fats raise blood cholesterol and triglyceride levels. They are primarily found in animal and dairy products, such as meat, egg yolks, milk, butter, cheese, cream and a few vegetable fats, such as coconut oil, palm oil and hydrogenated vegetable shortenings. Saturated fats are generally hard or solid at room temperature. Fats are also present in fried foods, potato chips, creamed sauces, mayonnaise and pastries to name a few. Learn to read labels on cans and packages, looking for the fat content listed.

Polyunsaturated fats help to lower the levels of cholesterol in the blood and reduce the risk of high blood pressure. They are mostly derived from plant and vegetable sources, such as cottonseed, soybean, corn and safflower. Sunflower and sesame seeds, walnuts and pecans are also high in polyunsaturates. Polyunsaturated fats are usually soft or liquid at room temperature.

Monounsaturated fats, like olive oil, have been found to lower high blood pressure (*Journal of the American Medical Association* 257:3251-56). Increasing your monounsaturated fats while decreasing your saturated fats should help lower your blood pressure naturally.

The American Heart Association recommends that saturated fats comprise only 30 percent of total calorie intake; others suggest even lower levels of only 10 to 15 percent. These levels are substantially lower than the levels found in typical American diets.

Diets high in protein, as from meat, and low in lysine, as from low-fat dairy products, can contribute to heart disease.

Use these tips to help reduce your cholesterol level and lower your blood pressure naturally.

• Do not consume more than 100 mg of cholesterol for each 1,000 calories. Daily cholesterol should not exceed 300 mg.

• Saturated fats, found in red meats and dairy products, should be reduced to less than 10 percent of total calories. Foods that are rich in cholesterol should be avoided or drastically limited in the diet. These foods include egg yolks, organ meats and most cheeses. Foods that should be reduced because they are high in saturated fats include butter, bacon, beef, whole milk, cream, chocolate, almost any food of animal origin, hydrogenated vegetable shortenings, coconut oil and palm oil.

- Unsaturated fats, such as fish and vegetable oils, may constitute as much as 10 percent of total calories.

- Total fat intake should be less than 30 percent of your daily calories.

- Try to avoid artificial and non-dairy creamers. If you need to use a powdered product (due to lack of refrigeration), use low-fat powdered milk. The instant, non-fat dry milk is convenient and has a lower fat content than a non-dairy cream substitute.

- Cut back on beef, lamb and pork. Never eat any combination of them more than three times per week.

- Don't eat duck, goose or organ meats. They are high in fat.

- If you must eat beef, use only lean cuts. When cooking at home, cut off all visible fat. In an Australian study reported in *The American Journal of Clinical Nutrition* (50,2:280), men who ate very lean meat cut their total cholesterol levels by 5 percent, and they lowered their diastolic pressures an average of two to five points. (HDL cholesterol levels also dropped, but the researchers said these levels would stabilize over time.) Broil or roast the meat in its own juices instead of frying. When eating out, select the best quality cuts. Keep your portions small and don't use any gravy or sauce. Also, avoid casseroles and pies.

• When preparing chicken or turkey, be sure to cut off the skin because much of the fat is contained in the skin. Eat the light meat on a turkey or chicken because it contains less fat than the dark meat.

• When eating red meat, serve less meat by preparing dishes that use meat plus vegetables, pasta or grains. Then you can use less meat per person while still providing adequate protein, vitamins and minerals. Stir-frying strips of meat with vegetables or cooking them in a wok are good examples.

• For dishes that require ground beef, substitute ground turkey (without the skin).

• Don't buy meat, fish or poultry that is already breaded. If you want to bread the meat, make your own breading with plain bread crumbs, herbs, skim milk and egg whites. Don't deep-fry after breading.

• Avoid prepared luncheon meats. As well as being high in fat, they are high in sodium and nitrites. Sliced turkey breast, tuna salad and salmon salad (without mayonnaise) are good luncheon alternatives.

• When making soup, chili or stew, place the broth in the refrigerator overnight. In the morning, remove any fat that has hardened at the top.

• Eliminate bacon bits from your diet. In salads and soups, try homemade croutons or herbs to add that "spicy" taste.

- Limit your egg yolks to two per week. This includes not only whole eggs but eggs used in baking and cooking. To reduce cholesterol, *Cardiac Alert* (9:5) recommends using two egg whites instead of one whole egg in cooking and baking.

- If you are using egg substitutes in trying to reduce your cholesterol intake, be careful. Many commercial egg substitutes are high in sodium or high in fat, even though they may be cholesterol-free. The American Heart Association recommends making a cholesterol-free egg substitute especially for use in baking: Beat three egg whites. Then add 1/4 cup non-fat milk, one tablespoon non-fat dry milk powder, and one teaspoon of polyunsaturated vegetable oil. Mix these four ingredients together to make a healthful egg substitute.

- When buying pasta, avoid noodles made with eggs.

- Avoid crackers that contain lard or "animal fat." Study the list of ingredients and buy only crackers made with acceptable vegetable oils. If a cracker leaves a grease stain on a paper towel, it contains too much fat.

- Avoid croissants.

- Switch from butter to margarine, preferably soft margarine. People usually use less soft margarine because it is easier to spread.

- Don't use saturated fat like lard, shortening or animal fat drippings for cooking. Use polyunsaturated oil like corn, safflower, sesame seed, cottonseed, soybean and sunflower oils. Monounsaturated oil like olive oil is best for your health, according to recent studies. Polyunsaturated oils like corn, safflower, seasame seed, cottonseed, soybean and sunflower oils are better for your heart and arteries than saturated fat, but they are not quite as good as monounsaturated oils.

- Eliminate one pie crust when baking pies. Make your pies "open-faced" rather than covering them with a second crust.

- For sautéing, use a vegetable spray. The spray will limit the amount of fat you will use in cooking.

- Avoid butter or sour cream on baked potatoes. Eating a plain baked potato is good for you and low in fat!

- Substitute low-fat cottage cheese or non-fat yogurt for sour cream in your favorite recipes.

- Avoid avocadoes and olives.

- Reduce the amount of peanut butter in your diet or eliminate it entirely.

- Eliminate french fries, potato chips and all fried "fast food" from your diet.

- If you want cheese, eat moderate amounts of the low-fat varieties like Mozzarella, Provolone and Swiss. For the taste of cheese, try a sprinkle of grated Parmesan cheese. It will still give you a cheese flavor, but it contains fewer grams of fat.

- Avoid heavy salad dressings like blue cheese. Try to eat less salad dressing by placing the dressing on the side and using it only as necessary.

- Drink skim or low-fat milk. Avoid using whole milk; evaporated milk; or sweetened, condensed milk.

- Switch from ice cream to ice milk, sherbet, sorbet or frozen fruit treats. Beware of frozen yogurt, unless it is frozen low-fat yogurt.

- Limit your intake of baking chocolate or milk chocolate which contains highly saturated cocoa butter. Substitute cocoa powder for chocolate when possible in recipes. The American Heart Association recommends substituting three tablespoons of cocoa powder and one tablespoon of polyunsaturated oil for each one ounce piece of baking chocolate. It will cut the amount of saturated fat by over 60 percent.

- Try scallops. They are a low-fat, low-cholesterol seafood. Avoid lobster and shrimp.

- Avoid all foods prepared with sauces or gravies like a cheese sauce (described as "au gratin"), hollandaise sauce, lobster sauce, sweet and sour sauce, mayonnaise or regular gravy. Tomato sauce may also be high in salt.

- When buying processed foods, look for "catch words" on the label that indicate high-fat or high-cholesterol levels: lard, butter, shortening, fat, cream, hydrogenated or hardened oils, palm, palm kernel oil, coconut oil, whole-milk solids, whole-milk fat, egg solids, egg-yolk solids, animal fat, animal byproducts, cocoa butter, milk chocolate or imitation milk chocolate. Avoid these products.

- Check food labels very carefully. Products labeled "low-cholesterol" may not conform to the same standards and could be high in saturated fats.

- Eat chick-peas, soybean products, oats and carrots to help maintain low cholesterol levels. Oat bran is an excellent source of water-soluble fiber and can reduce blood cholesterol levels by six to 19 percent, based on data from the Lipid Research Clinic in Illinois. Researchers at Northwestern University (*Journal of the American Dietetic Association*) discovered that about two cups of oatmeal or two oat bran muffins daily, combined with moderate levels of dietary fat and cholesterol, can lower cholesterol levels in just a few weeks. If you prefer oat bran muffins, be sure to use a low cholesterol substitute, rather than eggs, in the muffins.

For best overall health, also eat foods like fruit, bran, whole-grain breads and cereals. These foods may not lower cholesterol as well as oat bran does, but they are better than oat bran for preventing colon cancer and other diseases.

Omega-3

Most doctors don't recommend cod liver oil for their patients anymore because it also contains cholesterol. But, an increasing number of researchers and physicians are discovering the many healing benefits of that natural ingredient, now called omega-3 fatty acids by scientists and simply "fish oil" by the rest of us, which includes lowering blood pressure levels.

The insides of arteries suffer injuries, sometimes from turbulent blood flow. Sticky platelets in the blood collect around the injured area and send chemical signals for more sticky helpers, including germ-fighting white cells. The result, sometimes, is too much help.

Cholesterol, a natural part of blood, collects in unusual amounts at the growing bottleneck in the busy blood pipeline. The "helpers" continue to send signals that cause more of the blood's clotting agents to pile on the growing mass. The result is atherosclerosis, a form of hardening of the arteries, caused by fatty plaque growing on and changing the walls inside arteries.

These plaque blockages reduce blood flow, especially in arteries feeding the heart. Reduced blood flow, in turn, starves whole areas of heart muscle, resulting in heart pain (angina) or even heart attacks. Plaque blockages also cause blood clots to form, further reducing blood flow. That can happen in many areas of the body besides the heart.

And healing apparently is what omega-3 does inside blood vessels. Omega-3 fish oil helps the healing process by making the blood helpers less sticky and by keeping them from piling up and blocking the artery.

It helps in a second way, too. One part of the fish oil, EPA (eicosapentaenoic acid), gets into the cells that make up the artery walls. The EPA-fortified cells start cranking out their own chemical signals that order sticky. clot-forming platelets to stay away.

Recent studies suggest that fish oil taken before and after two very different kinds of surgery can have highly beneficial effects. In one study, fish oil seemed to help keep arteries unclogged after "balloon" surgery. In another, fish oil apparently helped prevent the spread of cancer cells that escaped after operations.

An extremely high intake of fish oil can "dramatically improve" the results of coronary angioplasty, popularly known as "balloon" surgery, according to one new study at the Washington Hospital Center. Usually about one-third of arteries opened with angioplasty get clogged up again with cholesterol and plaque within six months. But Dr. Mark R. Milner said his research suggests that taking large doses of fish oil for just six months can cut that failure rate in half.

Fish oil seemed to help patients after another kind of surgery, as well. A Harvard Medical School study suggested that highly purified fish-oil supplements helped prevent the spread of cancer cells that may escape during and after surgical operations to remove cancerous tissue. Dr. George Blackburn of Harvard, who's also chief of nutrition support at New England Deaconess Hospital, said the fish-oil supplements were given to cancer patients a week before surgery. Following surgery, the patients continued taking the fish oil for three to six months. Blackburn noted lower rates of cancer spread, known as metastasis, in those who took fish oil.

Both doctors have a very conservative approach to fish-oil therapy for all but these two classes of surgery patients. Milner advised against taking fish-oil capsules for any other reason because, he said, the long-term effects are still unknown. "I never give fish-oil supplements to any of my patients unless they are having coronary angioplasty," he said. Blackburn recommended eating deep-water fish four or five times a week, rather than taking fish-oil capsules. In the fish-oil study on heart patients, 194 persons were randomly assigned to two groups following successful angioplasty. One group took nine fish-oil capsules per day for six months after the procedure. Each capsule contained a total of 4.5 grams of omega-3 fatty acids. That's about the daily equivalent of the fish oil in two cans of sardines.

The other group got no fish oil, but patients in both groups were told to eat low-fat, low-cholesterol diets. Both groups received the same post-operative therapy. Nurses trained in diet therapy called each patient monthly to provide counseling and to evaluate if the patients were sticking to their strict diet.

"Dietary compliance was equally good in both groups of patients," Milner noted. "They really tried to stick with a strict low-cholesterol diet." Patients' cholesterol intake was restricted to 100 mg per day, and dietary fat was limited to 25 percent of their total calories. By the end of six months, 35.4 percent of people who didn't take the fish oil showed signs that their dilated heart arteries had narrowed again. However, the recurrence rate in the fish-oil group was only about 19 percent, Milner reported.

During the study, eleven patients stopped taking the high doses of fish oil because of disagreeable, but not dangerous, side effects, including gas and other mild digestive problems. Milner said that most patients were willing to tolerate the side effects in order to possibly lower their risk of having a repeat angioplasty or needing bypass surgery.

Coronary angioplasty is less invasive than heart bypass surgery because it does not involve cutting open the chest cavity. Instead, the surgeon cuts into a leg or arm artery and inserts a catheter with a tiny balloon on the tip. He threads the narrow catheter through the circulatory system until its tip reaches the portion of the heart artery that is narrowed by fatty "plaque." Then the doctor inflates the balloon, squashing the plaque against the artery wall and enlarging the inner diameter of the blood vessel. Several blockages can be opened during the procedure. Since the use of angioplasty began more than a decade ago, scientists have been searching for a drug to reduce the procedure's failure rate.

Aspirin has proven to be helpful in reducing the number of heart attacks that happened during or soon after angioplasty. But aspirin doesn't seem to make a significant difference in reducing the six-month reclogging rate, known as "restenosis," said Milner, who is assistant professor of medicine at George Washington University.

Milner's findings are similar to the results of a smaller study of 82 patients at the Dallas VA Medical Center, reported in *The New England Journal of Medicine*. Milner said several research teams are doing comparable studies to confirm these results.

Fish oil seems to suppress the inflammatory response that follows an injury, Milner said. In angioplasty, the inner wall of the artery is sometimes injured by the balloon catheter. If the injured area heals rapidly, excess inflammation, scar tissue and blood clots may combine to clog the artery again. Fish oil seems to slow the unwanted speedy healing process and to prevent the inflammation and scarring. It also seems to reduce the tendency of blood platelets to form clots at the once-clogged site.

The outer membranes of almost all cells contain oils called omega-6 fatty acids. "Overdosing" patients with fish oil high in omega-3 fatty acids alters their cell membranes. Omega-6 fatty acids in the membranes are replaced by omega-3 fatty acids. This change seems to make cell membranes less "reactive," Milner said. Thus, a person whose cell membrane content is high in omega-3 fatty acids may have white blood cells that are slower to cause inflammation and red blood cells that are slower to form clots, both good effects for heart health.

Increasing fish oil in the diet helps to lower cholesterol (the harmful LDL type), and it can also reduce high blood pressure, reports Dr. Alexander Leaf, writing in *Your Good Health*, a publication of Harvard Medical School.

But that's not all. Other studies suggest fish oil helps the joints, cuts down on arthritis discomfort, and prevents or reduces the pain of migraine headaches (*Total Nutrition Guide*, Bantam Books).

More recent animal studies (*Science News* 134:228) indicate that well-fed mice on high-fat diets that included fish oils rich in omega-3:

- Lived twice as long as normal mice

- Had half the normal levels of harmful autoimmune responses (inflammatory diseases like rheumatoid arthritis and lupus, in which antibodies attack the body's own tissues)
- Showed a complete absence of kidney disease, which normally strikes all these kinds of test animals
- Had blood cholesterol levels half that in normal mice, even lower than those in another study group of mice that had been fed calorie-restricted, low-fat diets

Although you can get fish-oil supplements (usually sold as omega-3 in capsule form), many doctors say a safer way is to forget the pills and eat fish containing the oils. Eating fish avoids two common, unpleasant side effects of taking fish oil capsules — a bad aftertaste and burping.

The highest levels of the two kinds of beneficial fish oil ingredients (EPA and DHA fatty acids) are found in fresh or frozen fish that normally live in deep, cold waters.

Eating canned fish is not recommended, since the canning process destroys most of the omega-3 oil.

Best of the saltwater breeds are mackerel (Atlantic, king and chub), Pacific and Atlantic herring, European anchovies, chinook salmon, sablefish, sturgeon, tuna and mullet.

Cod is a cold-water fish, but it has relatively little omega-3 oil in its flesh. Instead, the cod stores omega-3 in its liver. But many doctors advise against a regular supplement of cod liver oil, since too much can cause overdoses of vitamins A, D and E.

Among freshwater fish, highest omega-3 levels are found in lake trout and whitefish. Shellfish like lobster, crab and shrimp have smaller amounts of omega-3, as do mollusks like scallops and clams.

Don't like fish that much? You can still get some omega-3 through plant sources, according to *Everyday Health Tips* (Rodale Press). But, most plants generally are lower in omega-3 than the same amounts of fish. However, there are exceptions.

For example, oat germ is a good source of omega-3, better than all but 15 kinds of oil-rich fish. Three and one-half ounces of oat germ have more omega-3 than the same amount of sockeye salmon or mullet.

Common dry beans have more omega-3 than ocean perch, Pacific halibut, red snapper and many other kinds of fish. The lettuce-like purslane, used in soups and salads in Mediterranean countries, is high in EPA. Also good are tofu, walnuts, wheat germ oil, several kinds of beans, soybean products and rapeseed oil.

Margarine also is a rich source of omega-3, largely because it's made from soybeans. Unfortunately, it also has more saturated fats than fish or other plant sources of omega-3.

Based on an uncooked serving size of 100 grams (approximately three and one-half ounces), the following kinds of fish are highest in total omega-3 fatty acids content.

Food	Total fat in grams	Total omega-3 fatty acids in grams
Atlantic mackerel	13.9	2.6*
Chub mackerel	11.5	2.2
King mackerel	13.0	2.2
Lake trout	9.7	2.0
Japanese horse mackerel	7.8	1.9
Pacific herring	13.9	1.8
Atlantic herring	9.0	1.7
Bluefin tuna	6.6	1.6
Albacore tuna	4.9	1.5
Sablefish	15.3	1.5
Chinook salmon	10.4	1.5
Atlantic sturgeon	6.0	1.5
Lake whitefish	6.0	1.5
European anchovy	4.8	1.4
Atlantic salmon	5.4	1.4
Round herring	4.4	1.3
Sockeye salmon	8.6	1.3
Sprat	5.8	1.3
Bluefish	6.5	1.2
Mullet	4.4	1.1

*About one-tenth of one ounce

Source — U.S. Department of Agriculture, Human Nutrition Information Service

The following are plant sources high in omega-3 fatty acids. The comparisons are based on a serving size of 100 grams (approximately three and one-half ounces).

Food	Total fat in grams	Omega-3 in grams	Omega-3 % of fat
Rapeseed oil	100.0	11.1	11.1
Walnut oil	100.0	10.4	10.4
Wheat germ oil	100.0	6.9	6.9
Soybean oil	100.0	6.8	6.8
English walnuts	61.9	6.8	10.9
Black walnuts	56.6	3.3	5.8
Tomato seed oil	100.0	2.3	2.3
Soybeans, sprouted, cooked	4.5	2.1	46.6
Dry soybeans	21.3	1.6	7.5
Oat germ	30.7	1.4	4.5
Leeks, raw	2.1	0.7	33.7
Radish seeds, sprouted	2.5	0.7	28.0
Wheat germ	10.9	0.7	6.4
Common dry beans	1.5	0.6	40.0
Navy beans	0.8	0.3	37.5
Pinto beans	0.9	0.3	33.3
Kale, raw	0.7	0.2	28.5
Spinach, raw	0.4	0.1	25.0
Strawberries, raw	0.4	0.1	25.0

Source – U.S. Department of Agriculture, Human Nutrition Information Service

In what may be the first such official argument, Norwegian researchers are suggesting that a minimum level should be established for "essential fatty acids," just as there are standards currently for vitamins, minerals and other basic nutrients.

Their suggestion is reported in *The American Journal of Clinical Nutrition* (49:290-300).

The Norwegian researchers, led by Kristian Bjerve, discovered that omega-3 fatty acids are essential for the normal metabolic processing of omega-6 fatty acids.

Omega-6 oils, close relatives of omega-3 oils, are found in things like safflower oil and other cooking oils.

The Norwegians found a direct relationship between daily doses of omega-3 oils and healthy levels of certain blood substances.

In their study, they found that 350 to 400 mg of omega-3 acids in the form of purified fish oil are needed daily to maintain normal plasma and lipid levels.

"Omega-3 fatty acids possibly also have some specific function in the retina (in the eye) and in the central nervous system," Bjerve says.

"Dietary fish oils are rich in eicosapentaenoic acid (EPA), a polyunsaturated fatty acid of the omega-3 series," according to *Postgraduate Medicine* (85,4: 406).

Essential fatty acids, like EPA, have been discovered to play important roles "in the control and prevention" of heart and artery disease, the lowering of high blood pressure and preventing unnecessary blood clotting.

Researchers are also investigating fish oil's potential to help in angina (chest pain), rheumatoid arthritis and other inflammatory disorders, kidney disease and breast cancer, *Postgraduate Medicine* reports.

High doses of fish oil lowered blood pressure in men with mild high blood pressure, according to a new study published in *The New England Journal of Medicine* (320,16:1037).

"We found that dietary supplementation with high doses of fish oil given for one month lowered blood pressure in men with mild essential hypertension, whereas a lower dose of fish oil, the same amount of safflower oil, or a mixture of saturated and unsaturated oils produced no significant change," reports Dr. Howard Knapp of Vanderbilt University.

The researchers compared the effect of the fish oil (15 grams daily, or slightly more than one-half ounce) with common prescription blood-pressure reducers. "The magnitude of the effect that we found was similar to that of propranolol or a thiazide diuretic in the Medical Research Council trial," Knapp says.

Although these results are promising, the researchers warn that "the clinical usefulness and safety of fish oil in the treatment of hypertension will require further study."

Another study at the Pennington Biomedical Research Center in Baton Rouge found that fish oil's anti-clotting action in animals "depends on the dosage of fish oil in relation to other kinds of polyunsaturated fats — not the absolute amount of fish oil consumed," *Science News* (135,12:183) reports.

"If confirmed in humans, the finding may lead to recommendations on how much of the different kinds of polyunsaturated fats people should consume," says the *Science News* report.

Since a daily requirement has not been set, and safe levels of fish-oil supplements have not been established, "the consumption of fresh fish two to three times weekly is likely a reasonable recommendation," says the *Postgraduate Medicine* report.

However, "deep-fried, smoked, overcooked, pickled and salted fish should be avoided."

Remember that processing also destroys some of the omega-3 fatty acid content, so fresh or frozen fish — the kind caught in deep, cold waters — are better sources of EPA than canned fish.

About three grams per day, or a little under one ounce per week, of omega-3 fatty acids is the best dose size for cutting levels of fat in the blood, say researchers in *The American Journal of Clinical Nutrition* (52,1:120).

In a Dutch study, researchers at Amsterdam's Free University Hospital tested the effects of four different dosages of omega-3 oils on several types of cholesterol and triglycerides, as well as on the germ-killing power of white blood cells.

The doses tested ranged from zero to six grams a day. It takes 28 grams to make one ounce.

Triglycerides are a form of fat carried by the blood. Scientists consider high levels of triglycerides to be a risk factor for heart disease.

They found that fish oil even in small doses reduces triglycerides and raises the concentration of HDL cholesterol.

The effect was dose-dependent, meaning that the more fish oil taken by the volunteers, the greater the benefits.

Up to a point, that is. The body seems to be unable to use above three grams of fish oil per day in a beneficial way.

Feeding the volunteers six grams per day had no more effect than giving them three grams a day, the researchers report.

Some people shouldn't take fish-oil supplements or eat higher than normal amounts of food containing EPA and DHA.

Those with diabetes, persons with a history of hemorrhaging or strokes, or patients facing surgery or on aspirin and blood-thinning therapy should avoid fish oil unless specifically authorized by their doctors.

Fish oil can decrease the blood's ability to form clots. In addition, some people report heartburn and belching as side effects of taking fish-oil capsules.

Check with your doctor before taking any omega-3 supplements.

Olive oil

Olive oil is good for more than tasty salads.

Studies show that olive oil provides double-barreled protection for your heart, reports the *Medical Tribune* (31,20:15).

Olive oil is rich in monounsaturated fatty acids, and these fatty acids can have two positive effects on your health.

- Lowers cholesterol. Your doctor has been telling you to avoid saturated and hydrogenated fats (usually hardened fats, such as cooking lard) because they can raise your cholesterol. However, olive oil is rich in unsaturated fats that can actually lower your LDL cholesterol level. (LDL cholesterol is the "bad" cholesterol.)

- Reduces risk of atherosclerosis. This disease begins as "scratches" on the inside of your arteries. This is similar to rubbing coarse sandpaper on the inside of a plastic pipe. These "scratches" are a good place for cholesterol to attach and build up.

The scratches can be caused by a chemical change (oxidation) in the LDL cholesterol in your blood. The olive oil helps keep the chemical change in the LDL from happening. This reduces the chances of "scratches" forming and lowers your risk of heart disease.

At Stanford Medical School, Dr. Stephen Fortmann has found that one tablespoon of olive oil per day equalled a 3.1 drop in systolic pressure. If three tablespoons of olive oil or other monounsaturated fats were added to the daily diet or substituted for saturated fats, the systolic pressure could drop up to 9.4 points, and the diastolic pressure could be reduced by 6.3 points, Fortmann claims.

So, stock your kitchen with olive oil. It's great in your salads, and it helps you protect a healthy heart.

Corn oil

Corn oil seems to be able to lower the level of plasma fibrinogen in the blood, reports the *Journal of the American College of Nutrition* (9,4:352).

Plasma fibrinogen is a kind of protein in the blood that helps make blood "sticky" and form clots. Too much fibrinogen causes the blood to "thicken" and clot abnormally.

Abnormal clotting is unhealthy and may contribute to strokes, atherosclerosis (hardening of the arteries) and heart disease.

Since some oils seem to lower the amount of fibrinogen, scientists wanted to find out which one does the best job: dietary fish oil, corn oil or olive oil.

They fed the oils to three groups of volunteers for eight weeks and then tallied the results.

The fish-oil group and the corn oil group were number one and two in lowering plasma fibrinogen. Olive oil was least effective and came in third.

Researchers already knew that fish oil lowers fibrinogen levels. But, what's new is the discovery that corn oil also does a good job in making blood more "slippery" and less liable to stick together in clots.

Corn oil might become the latest nutritional weapon against strokes and heart disease, the report suggests.

9

THE FIBER STORY

Diets low in fiber

With the knowledge gained from research in the last 10 years, you now have available to you a lot of health information that will help you make intelligent choices about what to eat.

Out of all the technical terms and information, here's one solid piece of nutritional advice — eat more fiber.

One hundred years ago, the typical western diet contained an adequate amount of natural food fiber. Most bread was made with whole wheat flour which contained bran, the outer fibrous part of the wheat kernel. Coronary heart disease was rare at this time, and few people were troubled with appendicitis, diverticulosis, cancer of the large bowel, constipation, hemorrhoids, diabetes, obesity or high blood pressure.

Then, in the last quarter of the 19th century, American industry made two discoveries which were hailed as breakthroughs. The first invention was the development of high-speed-steel-roller mills for flour milling. Food companies could produce a fine white flour which tasted better than most whole wheat flour and was less likely to spoil. The second development was the growth of the canning industry, and the canning process greatly reduced food fiber content.

These two changes took place over several years, and no one noticed that anything was wrong. But in the 20th century, scientists became puzzled at the persistent rise in certain death rates and obesity. Commentators noticed that people in less developed countries didn't suffer very much from these ills.

In the 1940s and 50s, Dr. Denis Burkitt, a British surgeon, noticed that he never found a case of diverticular disease or cancer of the colon in the thousands of rural tribesmen of East Africa that were autopsied. Further research showed that obesity, appendicitis, heart attacks, constipation and hemorrhoids were also extremely rare. Dr. Burkitt thought that the amount of fiber in the diet was the key. He, and other doctors like Cleave, Trowell and Heaton, investigated what happened to tribes who moved to African cities and adopted a typical, low-fiber western diet. The results confirmed the hypothesis. On a diet that had been depleted of bran and other fiber, many Africans became obese and developed all the other ills of western civilization (*Journal of the American Medical Association* 229:1068-74). Dr. Burkitt also linked high blood pressure with a lack of fiber in the diet (*JR College of Physicians* 9:138-46).

Many brans give you what's called insoluble fiber. That's the kind that passes through your digestive system pretty much unchanged from the way it went in your mouth.

As its name suggests, soluble fiber is able to dissolve in water. When soluble fiber gets to the intestines, it actually swells as it rapidly soaks up water.

While most of us generally lump all soluble fibers into one big category, researchers are a little more specific.

The soluble fibers contained in oat bran include pectin, gums and mucilages.

These all have a well-documented ability to lower lipid (fat and cholesterol) counts.

When the insoluble fiber gets into the intestine, it dramatically reduces the amount of time food spends in the digestive tract. This reduces the possible harmful effects of wastes staying in the system longer than necessary.

This speed has its down side. Some minerals, such as calcium and zinc, may actually be bound by fiber. That means these important minerals have a harder time getting into the body.

These drawbacks should be dealt with, but they should not take away from the other important benefits which fiber contributes to the diet.

Soluble, dietary fibers have been shown to attach to and remove bile acids in the digestive tract. Bile acids are produced by the liver to aid in digestion.

The removal of these acids helps slow the development of micelles, which are necessary for the absorption of cholesterol and other lipids.

Fewer micelles mean less cholesterol and even less digested sugar can get into the bloodstream.

Soluble fiber contributes to good health by lowering the total amount of cholesterol circulating in the bloodstream, especially the LDL cholesterol. It also helps diabetics regulate their blood-glucose levels, leading to a reduction in the amount of doctor-prescribed insulin needed.

In one study, a group of 20 men with cholesterol levels over 260 were given diets containing 17 grams of soluble fiber per day.

This fiber was added to the men's diets from oat products and beans. This is equivalent to one serving of hot oat bran cereal and five oat bran muffins per day or several servings of cooked beans and bean soups.

After only three weeks on this high-soluble-fiber diet, the men averaged a 24 percent drop in LDL cholesterol.

While HDL cholesterol decreased slightly in this study, other studies have shown that HDL generally improves, or is not affected, when subjects start eating more soluble fiber.

In another study, both men and women were included in the research. These middle-age people usually followed diets that were fairly low in fat and cholesterol.

During the study, their already good diets were supplemented with two ounces of oat bran or oatmeal. This adds up to only 5.6 grams of soluble fiber for the oat bran or 2.7 grams for the oatmeal.

Even though this was a relatively small amount, these people reduced their blood cholesterol levels an additional 5 to 7 percent beyond the reduction they achieved by following their low-fat, low-cholesterol diets.

Other studies were conducted by Dr. James Anderson at the University of Kentucky.

In 1984, he reported that his subjects' high-cholesterol levels fell by 21 percent when they were given 3.5 ounces of oat bran per day for 21 days.

The same doctor also conducted a study at the Massachusetts Institute of Technology that compared oat bran versus wheat bran usage and their effects on cholesterol levels.

Students who ate 1.5 ounces of oat bran a day saw their cholesterol levels drop by 9 percent. Wheat bran had no effect on blood cholesterol levels, Anderson reported.

Keep in mind that a 9 percent drop in cholesterol readings for healthy college students cuts the likelihood of an early heart attack by as much as 30 percent.

Beyond the general description of the work of soluble fiber on bile acids, researchers are not entirely clear about just how soluble fiber produces all its benefits.

This is because so many different studies have been done, using different methods and different ways to examine the fiber.

However, many researchers agree that the benefits you will get from soluble fiber, including oat bran, is related to the amount you eat.

When a moderate amount of soluble fiber is eaten each day, a 10 to 20 percent reduction in cholesterol may be reasonably expected.

Oat bran

Oat bran provides the soluble fiber to help reduce high cholesterol levels and the heart problems they bring. And oat bran has the insoluble fiber to help prevent many types of digestive problems and cancers.

Oat bran may also be prepared in many tasty ways and may easily be incorporated into your everyday diet.

Oat bran is good for you for a number of reasons.

First of all, oat bran is readily available in fairly unprocessed forms. The less processing, the better it is for you. That means it will retain its important proteins, carbohydrates and vitamins B and E. Second, oat bran contains properties that help fight some of America's major killers. These include cancer, heart disease, obesity, high blood pressure and diabetes. Most specifically, it helps to fight high blood cholesterol, a condition that leads to a variety of health problems.

About half of the fiber in oat grain is soluble fiber. That leaves about 50 percent more in the form of insoluble fiber or roughage.

Insoluble fiber is not able to dissolve in water. It is the indigestible part of the foods we eat.

While it doesn't dissolve in the water in our digestive systems, it can hold and bind water to a certain extent.

Unfortunately, for years, this part of food was often labeled "non-essential." But researchers have gradually increased their recognition and respect of this part of our diet.

Beware of high-fiber claims in foods that are commercially prepared.

Many nationally-known companies began marketing "high-fiber" products when wheat germ became popular several years ago.

The recent emphasis on oat bran has created quite a stir, and food companies have begun selling all kinds of "high-oat-fiber" products. Many of these products either contain so little extra fiber or add so much fat that the good of the fiber is almost canceled out.

For example, you would probably say that a muffin would make a better snack than a cookie or that an oat bran waffle would make a better breakfast than a doughnut. But that's not always true. One company's oat bran muffin has more fat and more calories than a creme-filled doughnut.

Nutritionists at Tufts University set out to see what is good and bad in commercially prepared muffins. Some manufacturers were reluctant to say what's in their muffins. But through laboratory testing Tufts found:

• A simple raisin bran muffin sold through a national doughnut chain had 418 calories, 13 g of fat and 692 mg of sodium. (Keep in mind that it is usually necessary to eat several muffins just to get the needed dietary fiber.)

• A nationally-distributed grocery store oat bran muffin had 220 calories, 8 g of fat and 380 mg of sodium.

• An apple and spice muffin from a doughnut shop had 327 calories, 11 g of fat and 382 mg of sodium.

• Another doughnut shop offered a corn muffin. Its totals? It had 347 calories, 13 g of fat and 577 mg of sodium.

These figures should cast some doubt in your mind about the "healthy" muffins now offered commercially.

Your best bet may be to make your own oat and high-fiber

products. That way, you know exactly what is going into them.

Also, learn to read labels and ask questions. But be aware that lots of fat, cholesterol and calories could be hidden in the generalized information that you may receive.

A new study suggests that two to three ounces of oat bran added to the diet every day for about six weeks could reduce your cholesterol levels by 7 to 10 percent.

Funded by a grant from the Quaker Oats Company, a group of Chicago scientists tested the effects of oat bran on cholesterol levels in 140 volunteers, all of whom had high cholesterol, reports the *Journal of the American Medical Association* (265,14:1833).

The volunteers were divided into seven groups. All groups started eating a low-fat diet. Group one, the control group, ate one ounce of a wheat cereal each day, in addition to their low-fat diet.

Groups two, three and four added one, two and three ounces of oatmeal to their low-fat diet. And groups five, six and seven added one, two and three ounces of oat bran to their low-fat diets.

The seven groups stayed on these diets for six weeks. At the end of the six weeks, the volunteers tested their total cholesterol levels and their LDL cholesterol levels. (LDL cholesterol is the form of cholesterol that contributes to clogged arteries.)

Group one, the control group that ate wheat cereal, showed no drop in cholesterol levels. In fact, the group experienced a slight rise in cholesterol.

The group that ate two ounces of oatmeal daily experienced a drop of 2.7 percent in total cholesterol and a 3.5 percent drop in LDL cholesterol.

The group that ate two ounces of oat bran daily experienced a 9.5 percent drop in total cholesterol and a 15.9 percent drop in LDL cholesterol.

The oat bran had a greater reducing effect on the cholesterol levels than the oatmeal due to the oat bran's higher concentration of a kind of fiber known as beta-glucan fiber.

The study demonstrates that this type of water-soluble fiber, beta-glucan fiber found in oat bran and oat cereals, might be effective in lowering cholesterol levels.

The cholesterol-lowering effect is probably most effective when the oat fiber is combined with a low-fat diet, as in the study.

The study concludes that it requires three ounces of oatmeal to achieve the same cholesterol-lowering effects as two ounces of oat bran due to the higher content of beta-glucan fiber in the oat bran.

Anything less than two to three ounces daily results in fewer benefits, and anything more doesn't seem to do any more good.

Here are some guidelines for increasing your overall fiber intake:

- Make a good supply of bran muffins and keep them on hand for breakfasts and snacks and to serve as dinner "rolls."

- Eat plenty of fresh fruits. The old saying about eating an apple a day contains plenty of truth when it comes to increasing fiber intake.
- Try to reduce the amount of time high-fiber foods are cooked. Cooking breaks down some types of fibers and may slightly reduce the fiber content of the food.
- Avoid mechanical food preparations which ruin fiber in food before it is cooked. This includes peeling, mashing and grating prior to cooking. Instead, leave the peels on often-peeled vegetables, except potato peels which may sometimes contain harmful poisons. The peels not only provide fiber when eaten, they also add important vitamins and minerals. Cut fruits and vegetables into chunks rather than grating them.
- When given a choice, always select whole grains over more processed foods. More whole-grain breads are available, and cookies are now sold with less sugar and more fiber.
- When preparing recipes, try substituting whole wheat flour for one-fourth to one-half of the amount called for. Remember, if you are using oat flour, do not substitute it for more than one-third of the regular flour — it may interfere with the way things bake.
- Peas and beans are excellent sources of fiber. They have an added plus of being easily stored. Not only do they provide fiber, they are high in protein. They easily form the main dish at a non-meat meal.

- Try mixing mashed legumes into ground beef. This not only stretches the meat, it adds fiber and reduces the total amount of fat eaten. This mixture also makes a good base for Mexican-style dishes.
- Sprinkle oat bran and wheat bran on cereals, vegetables, desserts and even ice cream.

Rice bran

Oat bran and wheat bran aren't the only brans you should be eating. New studies have shown that rice bran is more effective than wheat bran in providing bulk and protecting against colon cancer. Like oat bran, rice bran is also effective in lowering total cholesterol.

Rice bran is "nutritious, has a light, slightly sweet taste, is a good source of protein and iron, and yet is low in calories and sodium," says Doug Babcock in *Cereal Foods World* (32,8: 538). In addition, it causes few allergic reactions, and it is easily digestible, he said.

Rice is also cholesterol-free and "contains only a trace of fat," explains *Consumer News* from Cornell University. "Rice is an excellent source of complex carbohydrates and provides thiamine, niacin, riboflavin, iron, calcium, fiber, phosphorus and protein," *Consumer News* continued.

"It has long been known that the bran layers of the rice kernel contain the highest concentration of nutrients," Babcock notes. "To gain the most food value, brown rice, which contains the bran layers, was the obvious choice. In fact, until recently, that was the only way we could enjoy the benefits of rice bran."

Now stabilized rice bran is available separately and can be added to your daily diet.

Lowering blood pressure

Fiber supplements were given to people in one recent study, reported by Danish researchers in *The Lancet* (2,8559:622-3). The people in the study discovered that their systolic pressure dropped an average of 10 points, and the diastolic pressure dropped an average of five points in just three months. However, people in the study who took a placebo (a harmless, fake supplement) did not experience a change in their blood pressures.

The National Cancer Institute recommends 30 grams of fiber each day. Fiber-rich foods include wheat and oat bran, fruits and vegetables (with skin), and whole-grain bread and cereals. When choosing a fiber supplement, like psyllium, watch for the sodium content.

Don't overdo it! A 75-year-old man must have thought, if a little oat bran is good, a lot is better.

After he suffered a week without bowel movements, increasing abdominal pain and frequent vomiting, surgeons at a Connecticut hospital opened up his lower intestine and found a 2-foot-long plug of "vegetable matter" that completely blocked his small bowel, according to a report in *The New England Journal of Medicine* (320,17:1148).

A week before he had to check into the hospital, the man had begun eating 60 grams (a little over two ounces) a day of oat bran in the form of oat bran muffins.

Six years before that, the man had part of his intestine removed because of diverticulitis.

Some inside scars from that operation, along with the "excessively high dose" of oat bran and the suddenness of the high dose without any gradual increase, probably caused the man's problem, the doctors speculate.

"We suggest that caution be exercised in the prescription of large doses of bran for the patient who has had abdominal surgery," the doctors advise.

A daily maximum intake of between 10 to 25 grams (under one-half ounce up to just under one ounce) would be better for people with past surgeries or other digestive tract problems, the report says. They advise a low-dose, breaking-in period first.

10

OTHER DIETARY FACTORS

The effects of alcohol

The relationship between high blood pressure and alcohol is well documented. Alcohol makes blood pressure skyrocket because it damages the liver and kidneys and causes fluid build-up, says Dr. Arthur Klastsy at Kaiser Permanente Medical Center in Oakland, California. Klastsy found that one or two drinks a day didn't affect the blood pressure, but excessive drinking caused blood pressure to rise dramatically (*Annals of Internal Medicine* 98:846-848).

Researchers at Harvard Medical School recently confirmed that blood pressure in women was also affected by heavy drinking. If 30 to 34 grams of alcohol, the equivalent of two mixed drinks or three glasses of wine, was consumed daily, women increased their risk of developing high blood pressure by 40 percent. The risk jumped to 90 percent in women who drank more than 34 grams of alcohol each day, reports researcher Dr. Charles Hennekens.

A major new heart study agrees with the two-a-day limit. More than that amount of alcohol daily may also drain a vital nutrient, calcium, from your body, says a report by the American Heart Association. That harmful effect shows up even if you take extra calcium supplements, the study indicates.

"Our study suggests that for the average person, at more

than two drinks a day, some bad things start happening physiologically," says Dr. Michael H. Criqui, co-author of the study published in *Circulation*. "Your blood pressure goes up, and you begin to lose the benefits of the calcium in your diet," Dr. Criqui says.

The study shows that non-drinkers and light drinkers who had higher calcium intakes also had correspondingly lower blood pressures, the AHA report says.

But, the study warns, those who averaged more than two alcoholic drinks a day suffered at least two bad effects. The alcohol seemed to raise their blood pressure, and the drinking seemed to prevent the blood-pressure-lowering effects of calcium.

Previous studies show that drinking alcohol apparently leads to poor absorption of calcium in the intestines, the report says. In addition, a heavier drinker passes a lot of calcium through the kidneys in urine, draining the body's stores.

Heavy drinkers sometimes have bones that appear to be "washed out" in X-ray photographs, because they lack calcium, the researcher says. That's added bad news for people at risk from osteoporosis, a bone-loss disease that strikes many women and some men over the age of 50.

You can't get around the bad effects of alcohol simply by taking more calcium every day, Dr. Criqui says. "We found that regardless of the level of calcium or potassium in the diet, alcohol still had an independent [bad] effect," says the researcher. "Alcohol seemed to be a much more powerful influence on blood pressure than either calcium or potassium."

The researcher recommends that you eliminate alcohol from your diet. Short of that, he says, do not have more than two alcoholic drinks a day. And because a diet rich in potassium and calcium may help reduce blood pressure, he suggests eating several servings every day of fruits and vegetables (containing potassium) and non-fat or low-fat dairy products (containing calcium).

Criqui and co-workers studied 7,011 men of Japanese descent who participated in the Honolulu Heart Study.

Another study found that older men and women were more likely to have their blood pressure increased by heavy drinking (*American Journal of Epidemiology* 118:497-507). The researchers were not sure if the increase was caused by a different reaction to alcohol in older people or if alcohol has a cumulative effect after many years of heavy drinking.

Estimates put the number of high blood pressure victims, as a direct result of alcohol consumption, at over 5 percent, and perhaps as much as 25 percent, according to the *Harvard Medical School Health Letter*.

Drinking just two alcoholic drinks per day can undo all the blood-pressure reducing effects of exercising, a new study at the Medical College of Wisconsin revealed. So don't exercise and then drink alcoholic beverages. High blood pressure that is caused solely by high-alcohol consumption usually disappears within a few weeks of giving up alcohol.

Taking garlic

For a long time, it seemed that garlic was popular with everybody except vampires and scientists.

For centuries, garlic has enjoyed great fame and popularity as a "miracle, cure-all" clove.

But scientists and researchers often dismissed the subject as simply another example of "primitive" folklore. Until now, that is.

Now, researchers are beginning to investigate the actual "powers" of garlic, and they like what they're finding.

In studies at the University of Vienna, Dr. F.G. Piotrousky discovered that garlic reduced blood pressure in about 40 percent of his high blood pressure patients, reports *Earl Mindell's Vitamin Bible*.

Other work at Loma Linda University has shown that four grams of garlic a day helped reduce blood fats in people with high cholesterol levels.

Garlic also seems to reduce the rate of heart attacks. Garlic eaters had 32 percent fewer second heart attacks and 45 percent fewer deaths from heart attacks than non-garlic eaters, reports *Science News* (138,10:157).

Another possible benefit of garlic compounds might be their "scavenging" effects.

Apparently, garlic increases the body's ability to remove substances in the blood that trigger cancer, says a recent study in *Preventive Medicine* (19,3:346).

Garlic actually seems to "clean" the blood.

So, eating more garlic results in much lower rates of

cancer, says the report.

For example, people in regions of China where average garlic consumption is high (a little less than one ounce per day) have lower rates of stomach cancer than people in the regions where garlic intake is low.

Since garlic can cause bad breath and body odor, *Earl Mindell's Vitamin Bible* recommends taking it in perles which dissolve in your intestines rather than your stomach. Researchers in Japan have produced another alternative called kyolic. *Prevention* magazine reports that kyolic provides the beneficial elements of garlic by lowering blood fats without the unpleasant side effects.

Caffeine

Caffeine can raise blood pressure significantly and should be avoided. A study in the *Journal of the American College of Cardiology* (53:918-22) found that men who gave up coffee had significant reductions in their blood pressure levels.

If you have a high-stress job, University of Oklahoma researchers say more than five cups of coffee a day can send your blood pressure soaring, reports *Modern Medicine* (57,11:22).

Thirty-four men took a simple test. They drank two glasses of grapefruit juice, one containing the amount of caffeine equal to that in two or three cups of coffee.

Their blood pressures were measured 15 minutes after finishing each glass.

Before the test, 17 men were identified at high risk for hypertension. Risk factors include diet and a parent with high blood pressure.

After drinking the caffeinated juice, those in the high-risk group had higher blood pressure levels than the low-risk group.

Other studies in *The American Journal of Cardiology* (53:918-22) have found that systolic and diastolic blood pressure levels were raised an average of nine points with just two cups of coffee.

If you're worried about your cholesterol levels or suffer from cardiovascular disease, take note. Research indicates that drinking one to five cups of caffeinated coffee every day nearly doubles your risk of heart disease and strokes, compared with non-coffee drinkers, according to *U.S. Pharmacist* (14,6:28). Six cups a day of the regular brew increases your risk 2.5 times, the report says.

A "safe" daily intake of caffeine is about 200 mg (less than one-hundredth of one ounce), according to the report. But one cup of coffee contains 100 to 200 mg.

Excess caffeine can provoke arrhythmia, an irregular heartbeat. That can be dangerous for some people. Too much caffeine also seems to be linked to increased levels of blood cholesterol. In one eight-week study, patients with existing heart rhythm problems got worse after taking the equivalent of three to five cups of caffeinated coffee each day, says a report in *American Family Physician* (39,6:214).

Researchers haven't managed to blame coffee for directly

causing cancer. But, they point out, heavy users of caffeine also tend to be heavy smokers. Tobacco smoking has been proven to be a direct cause of lung cancer. As for other cancers, "It appears that coffee drinkers are marginally more likely to develop bladder cancer than abstainers," says the *U.S. Pharmacist* report. A 1981 study suggested a link between caffeine and cancer of the pancreas, but that has not been confirmed in other studies.

Coffee is the major source of caffeine for most people. Just two cups a day can put you over "the safe limit," defined in this report as 200 mg. But did you know that a cup of percolated coffee has nearly 80 mg of caffeine more than the same cup filled with instant coffee? If you don't like decaffeinated coffee (which contains five milligrams of caffeine), try instant coffee instead to cut your daily intake, the report suggests.

Some other caffeine counts to note are the following:

Tea — 50 to 100 mg of caffeine per cup
Cola drinks — 33 to 50 mg per 12 oz serving
Cocoa — 2 to 8 mg per cup
Sweet, dark chocolate — 5 to 35 mg per 1oz serving
Chocolate desserts (ice cream, candy and puddings) —
   10 mg per serving

Note: Pain relief medication may also contain caffeine. One Excedrin tablet, for example, contains 65 mg of caffeine.

People who consume excess caffeine — 500 to 600 mg a day — might experience adverse effects such as restlessness, insomnia, flushed face, stomach upset, trembling, nervousness and irregular heartbeat. If you believe that you may be addicted, test yourself by not having your usual morning cup of coffee. If you have a severe headache later in the day, you might be addicted to caffeine. Such symptoms happen if you stop suddenly. Cutting back from large, daily doses of caffeine all at once might cause you to experience severe withdrawal symptoms, like throbbing headache, fatigue, irritability and anxiety.

Try to avoid "self-medicating" yourself with a cup of coffee. That's a step in the wrong direction, doctors say. Instead, try to cut down your caffeine habit gradually. If you're drinking three cups of caffeinated coffee a day, try to cut back to two cups for a week or so. Then cut back to one cup, and so forth.

Black licorice

Black licorice or licorice extracts should be avoided if you suffer from high blood pressure, according to researchers at Tufts University. Black licorice can make the body hold on to salt, lose potassium and cause fluid retention reports *The New England Journal of Medicine* (278:1381-3). People taking diuretics for their high blood pressure should be especially careful to avoid licorice because it seems to compound the problems and bad side effects of diuretic drugs.

Insulin

Insulin is a hormone produced by the pancreas, and it is needed to metabolize carbohydrates. When you eat, your body absorbs sugar and nutrients from the food and your blood sugar rises. Insulin is released and the glucose is either used or stored as glycogen, and your blood sugar levels go back to normal.

Insulin can be a significant factor in hypertension, according to a report in the *Archives of Internal Medicine* (152,8:1649). Researchers analyzed the results of 11 different studies conducted from 1983 to 1991. They found a definite correlation between insulin and high blood pressure, although it has not been proved to be a direct cause of hypertension. Besides controlling blood sugar levels, insulin also causes the kidneys to retain sodium, and scientists think this might be part of the reason why insulin has a bad effect on blood pressure levels.

Sometimes excessive amounts of insulin are released. People who eat a lot of sugary foods will produce more insulin. Overweight people may not be able to utilize insulin properly. So just cutting back on salt may not be enough. Watch your sugar intake, too.

11

LOSING WEIGHT

Obesity: How much weight are you making your body carry?

Study after study has shown that being overweight can put you at higher risk for high blood pressure. Also, the more you are overweight, the higher your blood pressure level will be. If you think about it, it's obvious. It is more difficult for the heart to pump the blood in an overweight person because the heart must pump more blood through more tissue.

Another problem for overweight people is insulin. Insulin is a hormone produced by the body and is necessary to metabolize carbohydrates. Often, overweight people have too much insulin in their blood, usually because their cells cannot properly utilize it. Insulin also causes the kidneys to hold on to sodium, and an excess of insulin means sodium retention, fluid build-up and higher blood pressure.

There are some overweight people who don't produce excess insulin, or they seem to be "immune" to the effects of too much insulin. For some reason, their bodies can handle it without raising blood pressure. But eventually time catches up with them, and their blood pressure levels do go up.

But how heavy is too heavy? Most medical professionals describe obesity as being 20 to 40 percent heavier than your ideal weight. However, health professionals warn that if you are 10 pounds over your ideal weight, you are overweight. About one quarter of the U.S. population is more than 20 percent over desired weight, according to the Centers for Disease Control in Atlanta.

And the heavier you are, the higher your risk of developing high blood pressure. Obesity is one of the major causes of high blood pressure, but studies also show that blood pressure drops significantly when weight is lost. By gaining or losing weight, you can affect your blood pressure.

Remember that measuring pounds is not the only way to determine who is fat. Body builders, athletes and people who do hard manual labor are often heavier than their "ideal" weight, but they are not overweight. Since muscle weighs more than fat, you can be heavier without being fat. If you can "pinch an inch," you need to lose weight. The pinch test can be used on the underneath of your upper arm or on your stomach. However, usually the pinch test is not necessary because most people know when they are overweight.

People with mild high blood pressure who lost just 10 pounds were able to stop taking medicine to control their blood pressure in a study reported in *Better Health* (5,8).

A second study involved nearly 800 overweight people with mild high blood pressure, according to *Medical*

World News.

First, researchers divided the big group into two smaller groups. They put one of the groups on a diet to lose weight, but the second group continued to eat normally.

Next they divided each of the two groups into three smaller groups and gave them either a diuretic, a beta-blocker or a placebo.

They found that people taking the placebo who lost 10 pounds or more had an average diastolic reduction of 12 points, about the same as those taking blood pressure drugs, the report says.

A different research team found a direct relationship between the amount of weight lost and the reduction in blood pressure. They found that with every seven pounds lost, the systolic blood pressure level will drop seven points and the diastolic will drop four points.

What is your ideal weight?

You probably already know what your ideal weight is. It's the weight at which you feel fit and healthy. You have plenty of energy and feel good about yourself. Your clothes fit comfortably, and you know you look your best.

However, there is an acceptable range of weight that depends on your height, sex and age. Most of us gain weight as we get older because our metabolism slows down, but as long as you are within the acceptable range, you are not considered overweight.

Acceptable Weight Range

Height	35 Yr	45 Yr	55 Yr	65 Yr
4' 10"	92-119	99-127	107-135	115-142
4' 11"	95-123	103-131	111-139	119-147
5' 0"	98-127	106-135	114-143	123-152
5' 1"	101-131	110-140	118-148	127-157
5' 2"	105-136	113-144	122-153	131-163
5' 3"	108-140	117-149	126-158	135-168
5' 4"	112-145	121-154	130-163	140-173
5' 5"	115-149	125-159	134-168	144-179
5' 6"	119-154	129-164	138-174	148-184
5' 7"	122-159	133-169	143-179	153-190
5' 8"	126-163	137-174	147-184	158-196
5' 9"	130-168	141-179	151-190	162-201
5' 10"	134-173	145-184	156-195	167-207

5' 11"	137-178	149-190	160-201	172-213
6' 0"	141-183	153-195	165-207	177-219
6' 1"	145-188	157-200	169-213	182-225
6' 2"	149-194	162-206	174-219	187-232
6' 3"	153-199	166-212	179-225	192-238
6' 4"	157-205	171-218	184-231	197-244

*Table values are for height without shoes and weight without clothes.

Source: Baltimore Longitudinal Study of Aging, conducted at the Gerontology Research Center, National Institute on Aging

What in the world are you eating?

Many times when you read about dieting, you are bombarded with information about calories, carbohydrates, fats and protein. What is even more confusing are the different ways these items are combined in different diets.

Sometimes diet books advocate reducing calories without saying which calories to reduce. Every day you could conceivably eat a hot fudge sundae and very little else. But what would that do to your health?

In the 1970s, low-carbohydrate diets were popular.

"Do not eat many carbohydrates," we were told, "but eat as many eggs and steaks as you want."

That was bad advice. A person may lose weight on such

a diet, but they could end up with arteries plugged full of cholesterol.

Who knows what weird combination will be advocated next, leaving many people just as overweight as ever and even more unhealthy because of an unwise diet.

Recent medical research suggests that you should eat more complex carbohydrates and fewer fats.

Just what are these carbohydrates, calories and other terms that all the diet people talk about?

• Calorie – Scientists would say that one "kilocalorie" is the amount of heat needed to raise the temperature of one kilogram of water one degree centigrade. In popular usage, however, the technical term "kilocalorie" has been shortened to the more familiar and more popular "calorie."

Thus, we use "calorie" to mean the amount of energy produced by food when utilized by the body. In other words, it is a way to measure the amount of energy that a food will produce in the body.

If a calorie is not used up during normal activity, it is stored in some form in the body for later use. If the amount of calories burned is consistently more than the amount of calories eaten, weight loss will result.

• Carbohydrates – These are energy-producing foods such as sugars, starches and cellulose. Carbohydrates are typically divided into two types.

The first type includes simple and double carbohydrates, such as honey and refined sugars.

The second type consists of complex carbohydrates, such

as the starches found in whole grains.

Simple sugars are easily digested and enter the blood-stream rapidly. This may cause difficulty for individuals who have trouble controlling the effects of sugar in the body.

In most people, simple carbohydrates will cause sudden peaking and dropping of blood sugar levels, which could lead to a craving for food and a net loss of energy.

Complex carbohydrates require prolonged action by digestive enzymes before the body can use the energy from these foods. The effects of complex carbohydrates on the body are much more gradual, and they are unlikely to lead to drops in blood sugar levels and overeating.

• Fats – For all their bad reputation, fats do play an important role in a healthy body. Also called lipids, fats are the most highly concentrated source of energy in the body. One gram of fat will produce about nine calories for the body's use (or storage).

Fats are also important because they are necessary for the body to utilize vitamins A, D, E and K, as well as calcium. They also protect vital organs and help to insulate the body from changes in the surrounding environment.

As explained in other parts of this book, too many fats in the diet will lead to excessive weight gain. Such an excess will also slow digestion. And too many saturated fats — the types that are solid at room temperature and usually come from animal sources — may lead to high levels of cholesterol and heart disease.

• Protein – This part of our diet is of vital importance for good health. Protein forms the body's "building blocks" for muscles, blood, skin, internal organs and hair. It is also necessary for both the formation and regulation of hormones.

When proteins are digested, they are broken down into simpler units known as "amino acids." The body can use amino acids only when they appear in certain combinations. These combinations are readily available in most meat and egg products.

The right combination may also be created by combining certain food products. For example, to create a complete protein using a food from the grain family (such as oats), it must be paired with a legume (such as peas).

But too much protein will lead to weight gain. Extra protein in the body can be converted by the liver and stored in body tissues as fat.

How can you lose weight?

Eat fewer calories and exercise. Most obesity is caused by underexercise rather than overeating, according to a recent report by the Department of Health and Human Services. The combination of exercise with a proper diet is important to fight obesity. These are very simple rules that can contribute to safe, gradual weight-loss. However, most people seem to want a "pill" that they can take so they will be thinner in the morning. Losing weight is a lifelong commitment to proper nutrition and regular exercise. It is not too difficult, although it may be a drastic change from a sedentary lifestyle.

Consult your doctor before starting any weight loss program especially if you are pregnant, over 60 years old and need to lose 20 pounds or more, or have an immediate family member who has had a heart attack or diabetes.

Here are some tips on how to change your eating habits so you can lose weight and keep it off:

- Avoid crash diets and dangerous weight-loss schemes. Choose a diet that you can live with for the rest of your life. Cycles of rapid weight loss, weight gain, weight loss and weight gain are extremely hard on the body's organs. Gradual weight loss that can be maintained is the healthiest way to lose weight.

- Before beginning your diet, write a list detailing your reasons for following a new eating pattern. Prominent on the list should be the health factors and reasons for wanting to lose (or maintain) weight. Keep the list handy for moments when you want to fall away from the diet.

- Keep a food journal of what, how much and when you eat each day. With a journal you can see exactly where your calories and nutrition are coming from and how you can alter your eating habits.

- Weigh yourself once a week and record it in your food journal. Daily fluctuations in weight are not reliable, but weighing yourself weekly will allow you to evaluate whether or not your program is working.

- Set a realistic goal for yourself, preferably with your doctor's endorsement. Being overweight is dangerous, but so is being underweight. Each person has a different metabolism that burns calories at slightly different rates. Choose a weight that is safe and healthy for your height, age and lifestyle.

- Choose specific times to eat your meals and snacks, and do not eat at any other time. Never miss meals because you may be so hungry at the next meal, you'll overeat.

- Do not eat if you are not hungry. As children, we were often required to eat "everything on our plates" and ate even when we were not hungry, but these patterns can lead to obesity.

- Learn to say "no" without feeling guilty. Once again, do not let someone force you into eating.

- Eat slowly. Put your utensils down after each bite. It takes several minutes for the stomach to tell the brain that it is full, so eating slowly will help you realize you're full before you overeat.

- Try to reduce your intake of all food rather than completely restricting yourself to certain foods. If you are not allowed to have a specific item, usually you will crave that "forbidden fruit." This is particularly true when working with overweight children. It is best to learn good overall eating habits rather than prohibiting certain foods for the rest of their lives.

- Drink grapefruit juice, unsalted (a low-sodium brand) tomato juice or unsweetened lemonade as an appetizer before your meal. If you allow 20 minutes before you eat, the acid in the juice will help you feel full, and you will be able to eat less. Drink the juice of a whole lemon squeezed into a glass of water, twice a day, for another natural appetite suppressant.

- Serve your meals on smaller plates so they will look fuller.

- Place the food on the plates away from the table. If you bring serving dishes to the table, you will be more tempted to have additional helpings.

- Never eat food out of the original container. Take out an appropriate serving and return the container to its proper place. By eating directly out of the container, you are more likely to eat too much.

- Try to leave something on your plate. In some oriental countries this is considered a high compliment because it shows that you have had plenty to eat. If you have been taught to clear your plate and not to "waste food," learning to leave a small portion on your plate will be good for you.

- Switch to lower calorie foods and calorie-reduced products. Always substitute skim milk for whole milk. Not only is this important for calorie reduction, it also is important for reducing animal fat in your diet. A one-cup serving of whole milk provides 150 calories and over 5 grams of saturated fat. Skim milk has 86 calories and less than three-tenths of one gram of saturated fat. Both non-fat dry milk and skim evaporated milk make good choices when cooking. Both have less than half of one gram of saturated fat.

- Many doctors now recommend avoiding products with artificial sweeteners. Although they seem to be a boon for dieters, some doctors believe that artificial sweeteners increase or maintain the desire for sweets which is not helpful to someone who is dieting. Using artificial sweeteners does not guarantee weight loss, reports research by the American Cancer Society. In a study of 78,000 dieters, people using artificial sweeteners gained more weight than people not using substitutes. The artificial sweeteners did not cause the weight gain. However, the researchers concluded that the people thought they were cutting back by using the artificial sweeteners, and they didn't limit their calories overall. Don't be lulled into a false sense of security — reducing total caloric intake and exercising are the only true ways to lose weight.

- Avoid diet pills, even prescription drugs, unless your doctor believes they are absolutely necessary. A 37-year-old woman nearly died when her heart stopped, Dr. Harry R. Gibbs reports in *The New England Journal of Medicine* (318:17,1127). The woman had been taking three drugs prescribed for weight loss. She didn't have any heart or artery problems. Gibbs warns that using inappropriate prescription drugs to treat obesity, even in someone without heart problems, can lead to "sudden catastrophic events."

- Do not use over-the-counter appetite suppressants. One common ingredient, phenylpropanolamine hydrochloride (PPA) has been found to cause high blood pressure even at the doses recommended for weight loss. Anyone with diabetes, heart disease, thyroid disease or high blood pressure should avoid products containing PPA, recommends the *Health Letter* (2:1).

- Do not use or purchase a product that promises to reduce or remove fat in one specific body area. Except for specific exercise or cosmetic surgery, one part of your body cannot be reduced.

- Do not use a "body wrap" in hopes of losing weight. The only weight loss that body wraps provide is the loss of sweat which is just temporary. Using body wraps can be harmful because they allow the body's temperature to increase.

- Eat more vegetables and smaller portions of meat, especially red meat.

- When you do serve meat, trim away any excess fat. Use the grill as much as possible so that some of the excess fat drips away during cooking.

- Always remove skin from chicken and other poultry before cooking. In restaurants, look for menu items that feature chicken that is baked or broiled without the skin.

- Eat plenty of high-fiber foods like whole-grain products, beans and vegetables.

- Use a low-calorie, soft-spread alternative to butter. If you use a soft-spread, you'll use less because it spreads easier than butter or margarine.

- Eliminate alcohol because it is high in "empty" calories. Alcohol products contain a lot of calories, but they have no nutritional value. Alcohol consumption is also a contributing factor in high blood pressure.

- Resolve never to consume calories in the things you drink, except for the calories in milk. Water, club soda, decaffeinated tea and coffee are all good no-calorie choices. Most soft drinks and fruit-flavored beverages are loaded with calories and have very little nutrition to offer in return.

- Switch from mayonnaise and egg sauces to non-fat yogurt and low-fat cottage cheese. The yogurt and cottage cheese can produce a creamy base for many sauces with far less fat and calories than mayonnaise.

- Before attending receptions and parties, eat a small, very-high-fiber meal. If you are full, you will be less likely to overeat. Plus, the high-fiber might help reduce your taste for fat-filled foods.

- Keep healthful snacks available. Try cutting up celery, carrots, broccoli, cauliflower, radishes and whatever other vegetables you like and leaving them in the refrigerator. Buy plenty of fruit. It provides quick and easy snacks.

• Reduce or eliminate high-calorie nuts and nut products, including peanut butter.

• Never go shopping when you are hungry. If you are hungry, you will be tempted to buy more, and you are more likely to buy high-calorie foods.

• Make a shopping list of things you need and stick to it. Don't be tempted by unnecessary foods.

• Make a habit of keeping food out of sight. Do not leave high-calorie snack food in the house. In the refrigerator, place raw vegetables and no-calorie drinks at eye level.

• Eat early in the day to achieve your maximum weight loss. Researchers at Tulane University found that people who ate their last meal at least eight hours before they went to sleep lost between five and ten pounds a month (*Postgraduate Medicine* 79:4,352). The participants did not change the amount of food they ate, or the number of calories, just the time of day it was eaten. If you eat most of your daily calories in the morning and at lunchtime and have a light snack for the evening meal, you should be able to boost your weight loss.

• The Good Wellness Program for Weight Management suggests placing a bottle of mouthwash in front of the refrigerator door. If you stray into the kitchen looking for "something to eat," you will have to move the mouthwash first. The director of the program suggests rinsing with the mouthwash to satisfy the cravings without consuming any calories.

- Brushing your teeth frequently may help reduce snacking. Your teeth and mouth feel so good that you don't have the desire to eat.

- Remember your diet when eating at a restaurant or some-one else's home. If you eat at a cafeteria, like a school lunchroom, check with the food services manager to see if low-calorie meals can be ordered.

- If you must have dessert, try sharing it with one or two other people. A small sample may satisfy your craving for a sweet.

- Serve a salad or low-calorie soup with most meals. They will fill you up, and you will eat smaller portions.

- Serve open-faced sandwiches. This will save you the extra calories of a second piece of bread. Always serve whole wheat bread.

- Do not go off the diet or stop exercising just because you do not feel entirely well. However, if you are truly sick, a day off from exercising might be a good idea. And if you have dramatically lowered your daily calorie intake, bring it back up to a less stress-inducing level.

- If you do break your diet, do not let guilt drive you away from your eating regime, even for a day. Read over your reasons for being on the diet in the first place, and pick up again where you left off.

• Never use canned fruit products that have been packaged in heavy syrup. Use fresh fruit or fruit that has been packed in its own unsweetened juice.

• Get out of the habit of watching television while eating meals. Sit down and really enjoy what you are eating, avoiding distractions.

• When flying or traveling by train, request a low-calorie meal at least 24 hours in advance of your departure.

• Do not reward yourself with food or use food to fight stress or depression. Buy yourself a gift or treat yourself to a favorite activity, rather than using food as a release or reward.

• Try squeezing your earlobe for one minute before eating. This is a technique of acupressure that may help curb your appetite.

• Obese dieters who lose weight very quickly are at increased risk of developing gallstones, physicians at the Cedars-Sinai Medical Center report. However, if four aspirin are taken each day, the dieter should not develop gallstones, according to the research. You should discuss the aspirin treatment with your doctor if you are considering a low-calorie diet.

• Exercise alone does not cause weight to "just disappear." According to a report in *The Physician and Sportsmedi-*

cine (18,7:113), you would have to walk about 22 miles to lose one pound. However, exercise is extremely important in helping you keep the weight off once you've lost it. Exercise should be viewed as a weight-maintenance tool rather than a weight-loss tool. It is fairly common for people who have lost some weight to gain it back simply because they didn't begin an exercise-maintenance program. On the other hand, those who commit themselves to an exercise program are usually successful in keeping the old pounds off.

Exercise helps some people lose weight because it increases their awareness of their bodies. Many people who start an exercise program are suddenly aware of what and how much they are eating. If you are faithful to your exercise program, you'll eat better and eat less because you won't want to "undo" the good your exercising has done!

Hazards of crash dieting

The sad fact is that the super-reduced-calorie diets — despite all their miracle claims — could set you up for a disaster, especially if you fall into a cycle of repeatedly gaining and losing weight.

In a Swedish study involving animals, Dr. Per Bjorntorp demonstrated that a body can actually become more efficient in gaining weight.

In other words, because of yo-yo dieting, the body might become super-efficient in turning calories into extra, unwanted weight. If that happens, you could gain more weight even if you eat less food and fewer calories.

That means you are less likely to keep weight off, and the next diet might prove to be more difficult.

Crash dieting or yo-yo dieting might also create serious health problems.

There is the possibility that the repeated weight-loss-and-gain cycle typical of a crash-dieter could encourage heart trouble or even a stroke. This has been suggested for two reasons.

First, yo-yo dieting tends to shift weight from the hips and thighs to the stomach. According to researchers at Boston University, a heavy midsection is linked to an increased risk of stroke in men and a high rate of heart failure in both men and women.

A second concern about quick weight loss and gain is the sheer stress this kind of dieting places on the body. This strain increases the risk of sudden death from heart disease.

If near-starvation is your idea of going on a diet, it is time to change your thinking.

Easy 'OJ diet' might help you lose weight

Scientists have discovered that water mixed with fructose suppresses your appetite better than glucose with water or even diet drinks. Fructose is the kind of sugar found in fruits. Drink a glass of fructose-rich orange juice half an hour to one hour before a meal.

You'll eat fewer calories during the next meal and still feel comfortably full, indicates a Yale University researcher in *The American Journal of Clinical Nutrition* (51,3:428).

The diet drink, glucose water and fructose-rich fruit juice all seem to work as appetite suppressants.

It's just that fructose worked better than sugar water. And the glucose water worked better than drinks flavored with a low-calorie sweetener. Plain water was least effective of the four.

In the fructose part of the study, overweight men ate nearly 300 fewer calories at lunchtime. Overweight women consumed an average of 431 fewer mid-day calories.

Their intakes were compared with similarly overweight men and women who drank plain water before lunch.

Even when the participants switched drinks, the results were the same. The new participants drinking the fructose-sweetened lemonade ate fewer calories than those drinking the other lemonade-flavored mixtures.

But what about the calories in the fructose drink itself? You might well ask.

Since the fructose drink was about 200 calories, the net calorie suppression was about 100 to 230 calories per meal.

That still puts the orange juice diet ahead of its glucose, diet drink and plain water competition.

If only for one meal, that still adds up to a savings of 700 calories a week or 36,400 calories a year, certainly enough to make a difference over the long run.

Long-term, slow weight loss is the healthiest form of weight loss for most people.

The diet benefit, however, doesn't carry over to soft drinks sweetened with high-fructose corn syrup. People who drank a lot of diet drinks reduced their intake of calories from sugar more than those who gulped regular soft drinks, says a report three months later in *The American Journal of Clinical Nutrition* (51,6:963).

Maybe you are carrying around an extra 10 pounds that keep your clothes from fitting just right. Or maybe an extra 30 pounds have accumulated over the years.

The point is, you want to be rid of the extra weight, permanently. First, the good news. You can lose weight, even if other diets have failed.

What's more, you don't have to starve yourself. In fact, popular sudden-weight-loss diets can cause you far more harm than good.

Even worse, crash diets might eventually make it even more difficult for you to lose weight.

However, before starting any diet, even a moderate-reduction diet, ask your doctor to make sure it's okay.

Some people such as pregnant women or people with certain diseases shouldn't try to lose weight.

Caution on the 'grapefruit diet'

It took three months of vitamin and mineral treatment to help a 47-year-old New York woman recover from diet-caused anemia, fatigue, leg swelling and abdominal pains and bloating.

She had used the so-called grapefruit diet for two years

and had lost about 50 pounds, but her health had faded during the process, according to a doctor's report in *The Journal of the American Board of Family Practice* (2,2:130). She had been eating unrestricted breakfasts, dinners and snacks but nothing for lunch except a grapefruit.

Her doctor found that she suffered from anemia, caused by an iron deficiency, and a severe deficiency of vitamin B12. The doctor put the woman in the hospital and gave her a blood transfusion. For the next three months, the doctor put the woman on a nutritious diet with the addition of a multivitamin supplement, one milligram of folic acid by mouth daily, iron sulfate by mouth twice a day, and monthly injections of B12.

A year later, the woman was still eating balanced, nutritious meals; had regained her energy; and had kept her weight to within five pounds of what she weighed when she first saw the doctor, the report said. What she discarded, the doctor said, was the grapefruit diet.

Diet and exercise teamwork

Dieting lowers your metabolic rate, or the rate at which you burn off calories, and exercise boosts your metabolic rate back to normal. Thirty minutes of daily exercise can burn off 150 to 200 extra calories a day, says *Stay Healthy* (3,12:46). According to the *Good Health Bulletin* (II,3:2), regular exercise also keeps your heart healthy by producing an enzyme that breaks down fats in the bloodstream. More on exercise in the next chapter.

12

EXERCISE

Exercise for your heart

A recent medical study praises the benefits of exercise in controlling cases of mild high blood pressure.

At the same time, the study suggests that adding drugs to the exercise program might be just a waste of time, at least in mild cases.

The natural way does the job as well as or better than high blood pressure drugs, according to a report in the *Journal of the American Medical Association* (263,20:2766).

In the *JAMA* report, doctors at three Maryland clinics studied three groups of men with high blood pressure averaging 145/97 mm Hg. None of the men exercised regularly.

They put one group on a beta-blocker; a second group on a calcium-channel blocker; and the third group received only a placebo, a fake, harmless pill with no medical effect.

All three groups performed the same kinds of exercises.

Three times a week, all 49 men lifted weights for 30 minutes on a 20-station weight-training circuit. Then they performed 20 minutes of aerobic exercises, either stationary cycling, walking or jogging.

After 10 weeks, average blood pressure had fallen 14 points systolic and 13 points diastolic to 131/84, the report says.

More significantly, the drop occurred whether or not the men were taking blood pressure medicine.

Exercise alone accounted for the improvement, the researchers conclude.

In addition, the men experienced a drop in total cholesterol and LDL cholesterol levels.

Levels of HDL cholesterol increased with the calcium-channel blocker but actually decreased with the beta blocker.

As added benefits, the men lost a little weight and increased their overall strength by an average of 25 percent.

Blood pressure varies with the condition of the heart. Exercise which increases the strength of the heart may help to prevent or lower high blood pressure. In addition to lowering blood pressure, exercise can also help fight obesity, constipation, osteoporosis and insomnia; increase mental alertness; help you cope with stress; increase your self-esteem; and reduce depression.

Since the heart is a muscle, it must be exercised like any other muscle to become stronger. If it is exercised regularly, its strength increases. If not, it becomes weaker. Although it is often believed that strenuous work harms the heart, scientific research has found no evidence that regular, progressive exercise is harmful for the normal heart.

A strong heart muscle can pump a greater amount of blood with fewer strokes per minute. For example, the average individual has a resting heart rate of between 70 and 80 beats per minute, while a trained athlete may have a resting heart rate in the low 50s or even in the 40s.

Before starting an exercise program consult your doctor and follow a recommended plan. Remember to slowly increase the intensity and duration of exercise. Don't overdo it in the beginning. Watch for body signals, such as sharp pains and cramps, that tell you when you're doing too much.

Regular aerobic exercise, at least 30 consecutive minutes three times a week, is the key to better fitness. Aerobic exercise increases your endurance, helps improve circulation and strengthens the heart. Spurts of activity can actually be harmful to a non-active person, so regularity is important. Swimming, cycling, rowing, skiing, jumping rope and aerobic dancing are some of the many aerobic activities that you can choose.

Anaerobic exercises, such as weight lifting and tennis (unless it's very vigorous), should be avoided. These exercises consist of short spurts of activity and do not "exercise" the heart, but they do raise the blood pressure and can be harmful if continued over long periods of time.

The *Journal of the American Medical Association* (212:2267) says that people with high blood pressure should avoid isometrics. Isometrics are exercises that involve muscle contractions while the joints remain in place, like squeezing the hand against a fixed object such as a tennis ball. In the *Journal*, Dr. William S. Breall warns that isometrics can cause a temporary rise in blood pressure which can be extremely dangerous for people with blood pressure that is already high.

Walking is the number one form of exercise, and it is usually recommended by physicians as the best exercise for people who are just getting started. Walking can help lower high blood pressure and improve your fitness level. If walking does not challenge you anymore, but you would like to continue, carry handweights. Small handweights, no more than five pounds per hand, will add to the upper body workout when walking and make your walk more beneficial.

Sports physicians are now recommending exercise that includes use of both the legs and the arms, according to *Physician and Sportsmedicine* (14:5,181). Window washers, farmers and orchestra conductors, all people who use their arms daily, seem to have an increased life expectancy. For a complete workout that includes the arms, try swimming, cross-country skiing or using a rowing machine. Before you start an exercise program, check with your doctor.

- Time. You must choose an activity that you are willing to devote time to every day or every other day. Set aside a certain time and stick to it. Let everyone in your family know that during that time you are unavailable. It's your time to do something for yourself.

- Pleasure. If you don't enjoy the type of exercise you are doing, you are less likely to make it a regular part of your daily life. Be willing to try several different activities. You may discover that a form of exercise you thought would be boring is perfectly suited to your needs and enjoyment.

- Variety. Don't be afraid to choose a variety of activities that you enjoy. You may discover that aerobic classes during the week and a long walk or hike on the weekend are a perfect combination for you.

- Success. Don't undermine your exercise by feeling guilty if you miss your planned activity. Look forward to your next time of exercise. Celebrate the successes you have enjoyed during your exercising. If you get discouraged, try doing the same routine or amount of exercise as your first time.

- Spouse. If you are married, having the support of your spouse can be very important. Finding an activity that you can do together can be great. Your spouse's support may make it easier for you to continue with regular exercise.

- Groups. Many people find that the support of a group makes regular exercise easier to continue. This doesn't mean you have to join an expensive fitness club or take a class. Just getting a small group of friends who are willing to meet and go for a walk on a regular basis can help. The companionship of the group, knowing you are not alone and enjoying exercise as a social activity are very helpful.

- Money. Some people find that a paid class is the best incentive for them to continue exercising. Even if you just have a little "miser" in you, you may feel the urge to attend all the classes because you don't want to "waste the money." If this works for you, keep paying for classes in advance!

When you're ready to begin exercising, there are a few things you must remember.

- Always do a few minutes of stretching exercises. If you don't warm-up first, you are more likely to be sore, and there is a greater risk that you will pull a muscle.

- Exercise for at least 30 minutes. Anything less is not really going to help your heart.

- Cool down. Never stop any aerobic activity suddenly. Slow the jog down to a walk. Get off the stationary bike and walk around the room. Do anything, but keep your legs moving until your heart rate has gone back down to normal.

People can find all sorts of excuses why they can't exercise. They don't have time, they are too unfit, they are too tired or they are too old. No excuses! Nobody is too old or unfit. Everyone can find 30 minutes sometime during the day. As for being tired, exercise gives you energy and makes you feel better. Do it for yourself and for your heart.

13

STRESS

How to cope

If you've ever suspected that your high-pressure job is bad for your health, you're probably right.

According to a study reported in the *Journal of the American Medical Association* (263,14:1929), men who hold jobs with high demands over which they have little or no control are three times more likely to suffer from high blood pressure than men who don't.

These workers are also more likely to suffer from physical changes to the heart that could lead to heart disease over time.

Researchers report that the risk of job-related hypertension increases with age.

Anxiety, frustration and anger may aggravate high blood pressure.

Being unhappy at work can raise your blood pressure, researchers at the University of Pittsburgh discovered. In a study of 288 men who had blue collar jobs, the researchers found that the more dissatisfied the worker was with his job, the higher his risk of having high blood pressure. If the man felt insecure about his job, had little opportunity for promotion, didn't feel part of the decision-making process or that the other employees were not supportive, he was more likely to have high blood pressure. Job stress and job dissatisfaction has also been linked to an increased risk of heart and artery diseases, reports the *American Journal of Epidemiology*.

However, many calm people have high blood pressure. Although it is a cause in some cases, you do not have to be under a lot of stress or be a "tense" person to have high blood pressure.

With "reactive" high blood pressure, the body reacts to stressful or threatening situations by releasing a hormone called renin from the kidneys. This prepares your body for "fight or flight," pumping adrenalin and speeding up the heart, sending more blood to the brain and muscles. It also causes sodium retention and elevates blood pressure. Some people naturally produce too much renin. These people usually have a "Type A" personality. They are competitive, agressive, tense, impatient and easily irritated. They also usually have high blood pressure. In some cases drugs are needed to restrict the production of renin. There is some evidence that low magnesium levels are associated with high renin production.

Learn to recognize your body's stress signals. Do you start to snap or lose your temper with loved ones? Are you more tired? Do unimportant little things start to bother you? Do you get headaches or body aches? Do you suffer from insomnia? Many of these symptoms plus clenched fists, chain smoking, biting your lips, sleeping too much, being quick to cry, and wanting to run away are all common signs of too much personal stress. The first step in alleviating stress is to learn to recognize its signs.

How can you reduce stress? It's impossible to completely eliminate emotional strain, but it is possible to avoid some stressful situations. Talking about a problem, working off your anger, making time for things you want to do, doing for others and learning to tackle one job at a time are only a few of the positive actions you can take to lower your emotional tension.

Certain events, both good and bad, are known to be stressful. Some of these events are planned and some are sudden and cannot be anticipated. Events that can cause stress include:

- Death of a spouse or a close family member
- Divorce, marital separation or reconciliation
- Personal injury or illness
- Marriage
- Getting fired from work
- Retirement

Whenever possible, try not to plan too many high-stress events at the same time. For example, getting married causes stress. If you buy a home, get married and start a new job all at the same time, you will be under a great deal of stress. However, if you can plan the events so they don't happen together, you can reduce your stress level.

Techniques for stress management should be appropriate for the kind of stress you experience. Physical methods like deep breathing and exercise should be used to cope with physical reactions to stress, like body aches, hyperactivity and nervousness. Mental calming methods should be used for mental stress.

Accept your own personal limitations. Accept the limitations of money. You will always want more than you have, and you may have to sacrifice some things to get what is important to you. Accept the limitations of your situation. If your plane is delayed or if you are stuck in a traffic jam, worrying and getting angry will not make the situation better.

Your approach to life has a lot to do with how much stress you create for yourself. For example, if you are a perfectionist about your own work and expect others to adhere to your high standards, you are setting yourself up for plenty of stress-filled days. Learning to accept things that are "less than perfect" could be important for your health. Even if you accept a few "less than perfect" projects, you will lower your stress. Also, remember your strengths and weaknesses. No one can do all things well. Try to improve your strengths and your weaknesses. Don't be too hard on yourself when you discover that you cannot excel at everything.

Cool your competitive edge. Rather than constantly comparing yourself to others, set your own goals based on your own performance. Don't be constantly trying to get the best parking space or get ahead of "that" car in traffic. Many times these minor competitions contribute to unnecessary stress in our lives.

Acknowledge your successes. Celebrate the things you accomplish, no matter how small. If you have a job that is repetitive, and it is difficult to see any progress, create and celebrate your own accomplishments.

If you always seem to be concerned with yourself, try reaching out to others. Doing something for someone else may help to put your problems into better perspective. Hopefully, you will become less self-centered as you appreciate the people around you.

Make time for yourself everyday. Do something that you enjoy.

Don't try to bear other people's stress. Learn to recognize that their problems are not your fault. You can be supportive and loving without carrying their stress.

Don't be afraid to get help. Asking for help is not a sign of weakness but rather a sign that you know your own limitations.

Don't be afraid to cry. Research has shown that crying is a natural and healthy way to deal with stress. Crying helps focus your emotions and provides a needed release.

Music is now being recognized and used by professional therapists to help relieve and treat stress. Music can change the breathing rate, the heart rate and the level of stress someone is experiencing. Music that causes you to relax will be most helpful. Songs from your past that you associate with good times can bring back those good feelings. Therapists prefer music without lyrics so you don't get caught up in listening to the words. After having a stressful experience, just lying down with your eyes closed and listening to the music should alleviate some of the symptoms of stress.

Music can also help prepare a person for a stressful situation. For example, if someone dreads going to the dentist or has an important business meeting, they can play their "calming" music on the way there. The right music can help you approach stressful events in a calm and serene manner.

If you have a stressful job, try to avoid bringing that stress home to your family. Taking your frustrations out on your family and friends may add to their stress. There is a place for discussing your problems with your family, and your family should be able to support you. But learn the difference between having their support and making them share the burden of your stress.

Talk. Share your concerns, your fears, your dreams and your anxieties to your closest friend or spouse. Talking helps put the problems into correct perspective.

Supplementation with vitamin C and iron, which is necessary for the formation of red blood cells which help carry oxygen to the body, may help fight stress. Stress may increase the need for niacin (vitamin B3) and thiamine (vitamin B1).

The best way to prepare your body to cope with stress is to get plenty of rest (seven to eight hours of sleep each night) and avoid eating high-fat or high-salt foods. Researchers in France, and Dr. Burton M. Altura of Brooklyn, New York, have discovered that low magnesium levels make it more difficult to deal with stress. Avoid cigarettes, alcohol, caffeine and any other substances that are harmful to the body.

Pharmacists are now claiming that certain fragrances can have a calming effect in times of stress. Many cosmetic companies are marketing fragrance vials that contain "spiced apple" or other smells that are supposed to help us relax. Research has proven that animals are greatly influenced by smells and aromas, but whether or not human beings can become relaxed just by breathing a certain scent is not known. However, if you have a certain aroma that you associate with peacefulness and calm, maybe fragrance therapy will help you relax.

Exercise can give you a chance to clear your mind as well as rejuvenate your body. Regular exercise will help improve your circulation, lower your blood pressure, and allow you to better cope with stress.

14

Smoking

Are you habitually damaging your heart?

Smoking is a well-known hazard to people with high blood pressure. Smoking cigarettes, pipes or cigars can constrict the arteries, which directly raises high blood pressure and increases the risk of heart failure. Many smokers continue smoking even when they realize it is bad for their health, because nicotine is a very addictive substance. It is extremely difficult for a smoker to stop smoking because of the physical craving for nicotine.

Smoking is a learned behavior. Human beings do not have a "need" for nicotine. To stop smoking, you must "unlearn" this behavior and break the nicotine addiction.

The American Cancer Society, the American Lung Association, Merrell Dow Pharmaceuticals and many other organizations have compiled these guidelines to help you quit:

• The desire to quit smoking will be your biggest asset when you try to quit.

• Examine your reasons for wanting to quit. Besides the physical damage of smoking, you may be helping your family and friends, as well as saving time and money. Write down at least 10 reasons for quitting. Review these reasons daily and keep adding to the list.

• Decide you want to quit. Be positive about your decision. Then choose a day to quit and stick to it. If you are a heavy smoker while at work, you may want to quit on a Friday afternoon. By Monday morning, you'll have two smoke-free days behind you and should be better prepared for the stress of your first smoke-free work day.

• Identify the times and feelings you associate with smoking. You may smoke after meals or while you are under stress. When possible, avoid the situations that you associate with smoking. If you feel the desire to smoke every time you have a cup of coffee or an alcoholic drink, cut out the coffee and alcohol as well. You may have to limit your social life until you feel secure about not smoking. Learning when you smoke and re-learning those activities without smoking can be the most difficult time in "kicking the habit."

• Organize pleasant and busy activities for the day you will quit. Plan to do things with other people, preferably non-smokers. Keeping an active schedule may help you get over the first few days. You may want to have some kind of treat or celebration to start your non-smoking campaign.

• If you are quitting "cold turkey," try to remove all temptations before you start. Throw away all cigarettes. Remove your ashtrays, lighters and matches.

• Keep your mouth clean. Brush and floss your teeth often so your mouth will taste clean. You may want to visit a dental hygienist and have your teeth cleaned within the first few days after you quit smoking. If you schedule the appointment beforehand, this appointment could be your first goal as a non-smoker.

• Some people find that sugar-free chewing gum helps keep the mouth occupied when you have the urge to pick up a cigarette.

• If you miss having something in your hand to play with, try substituting a pen or pencil.

• If you feel the urge to smoke, do something physical or take a bath or shower. Try doing more things with your hands, like writing letters, crafts, sewing, woodwork, housework or gardening.

• Maintain or improve your physical health. Start exercising regularly. Eat healthy meals, including lots of fruits and vegetables. Drink more fluids, including fruit juices and water. Everyone should drink at least eight glasses of water each day. Get lots of rest and relaxation. By getting your body in good condition, you will be better able to tolerate the physical symptoms of withdrawal from nicotine. Physical exercise will improve your breathing and blood flow, as well as provide a smoke-free activity.

• Get support. If your spouse smokes, try quitting together. You will be able to support and encourage each other. If not, involve someone else who will support you, and you will improve the chances of becoming and staying a non-smoker.

•Remember that smoking is not just a bad habit. Smoking is also an addiction to the drug nicotine. You may experience withdrawal symptoms. According to the Department of Health and Human Services, mood changes, irritability, aggressiveness, anxiety, difficulty in sleeping, drowsiness, weight gain, lower blood pressure, headaches, upset stomachs and a decrease in the heart rate are common physical reactions to nicotine withdrawal. Usually, the withdrawal symptoms subside within a few days or a few weeks. Withdrawal from nicotine might be eased by prescription drugs such as Nicorette, a chewing gum, and Nicoderm, a patch worn on the skin, by slowly releasing a measured dose of nicotine into the system to reduce physical craving. Withdrawal from nicotine may also be eased by taking 1/2 teaspoon of baking soda in a glass of water two or three times a day. Apparently, the baking soda helps hold nicotine in the system and reduces withdrawal symptoms by giving the body more time to adapt to withdrawal.

•While trying to quit smoking, *Earl Mindell's Vitamin Bible* recommends a variety of supplements to help overcome the withdrawal from nicotine. A good multivitamin, 100 mg of a vitamin B complex, 100 mg of cysteine and 300 mg of vitamin C will help keep the body healthy during the time you are withdrawing from nicotine, says Mindell.

• Don't try to have just one cigarette. Just like a reformed alcoholic, one cigarette can begin the smoking cycle again. Even in times of personal crisis, don't smoke.

• If you don't quit the first time you try, don't give up. Don't be too hard on yourself. There is a definite physical addiction to nicotine, and it may not be easy to quit. Some people need to try two or three times before they are successful.

• Accept the fact that not everyone can quit "cold turkey." Although this method may work for some people, it does not work for everyone. If you feel that the cold-turkey method is not for you, try cutting back on the number of cigarettes you smoke each day. Count the number of cigarettes you smoke in an average day, then smoke one less each day. You may need to count them every morning. Keep a chart and leave out only the number of cigarettes that you can have that day.

• If you find you cannot quit at this point, switch to a low-tar, low-nicotine brand of cigarette. But do not increase the number of cigarettes you smoke each day.

• Congratulate yourself with each step you take toward being smoke-free. Giving up smoking is hard. Be proud of yourself each time you give up one cigarette.

• According to Merrell Dow Pharmaceuticals Inc., "the risk of smoking again is the highest in the first few months" after you quit. Be careful and reward your achievements. Celebrate your anniversaries of non-smoking. Treat yourself after the first week, the first month and maybe every month after that. You deserve to celebrate.

15

ADDITIONAL INFLUENCES

Your spouse

Your mother always told you to marry the "right" person, but you probably didn't know how much influence your marriage partner can have on you. The disposition of your spouse or your partner's blood pressure has a great influence on your blood pressure levels. At the University of Texas, Marjorie A. Speers, Ph.D., discovered the relationship after examining over 1,200 couples, according to a report in the *American Journal of Epidemiology* (123:818-29). Other factors, like exercise, salt intake and obesity, were taken into consideration, but the spouse still influenced the blood pressure levels.

Your pet

Many health professionals are now recommending the loving companionship and responsibility that a pet provides. According to medical studies, in some cases having a pet can help people reduce their high blood pressure levels. Of course, pets are not for everyone. They require care which some people are not able to give.

Your conversations

Talking too much may irritate your friends, but did you

know it could also be hazardous to your health? Studies by Dr. James Lynch of the University of Maryland Medical School show that listening, rather than talking, lowers blood pressure. In a report in *Psychosomatic Medicine* (43:25-33), 98 percent of the 178 people studied had their blood pressure surge when they started talking.

The highs and lows of blood pressure levels won't hurt people with normal blood pressure, Dr. Lynch explains, but in someone with high blood pressure, the highs can be dangerous.

Dr. Lynch used an automatic blood pressure monitor and recorded continuous blood pressure readings during conversations with patients. In people with high blood pressure, talking about intimate problems raised their blood pressure to dangerous levels, according to Dr. Lynch.

Many people with high blood pressure do not speak normally, which causes their blood pressure to rise even further. Dr. Lynch claims that the louder and faster a person talks, the higher the blood pressure. People who emphasize their words, talk "breathlessly," use hand motions, interrupt or talk over someone else seem to experience the highest rise in blood pressure.

Dr. Lynch believes that slower speaking, combined with breathing more deeply and regularly during speech, helps to lower blood pressure. Anyone with speech-induced blood pressure problems can learn to speak more slowly, he says.

Learning to listen and focusing on what the other person is saying might lower stress and reduce the load on the heart.

Most people with chronic high blood pressure do not really "listen" to a conversation, Lynch explains. These people are so worried about how they will reply that they are defensive even when they are listening, and their blood pressure doesn't drop as much as it does in a person who truly listens.

In a University of Pennsylvania study, Drs. Katcher and Beck compared blood pressure levels during three different situations — while the participants just sat and did nothing, while they watched fish in a small tank and while they talked. The highest level was during speech, but the lowest level was while watching the fish. Being quiet isn't the key to lowering your blood pressure. You need to relax and focus on something or someone else.

Dr. Lynch believes that the most important thing his studies have shown is that "learning to listen to other people can help hypertensives lower their blood pressure."

The next time you visit your friends or family, listen to what they have to say. It will not only help them, it will also do your own heart good.

Your medications

Ask your pharmacist or your doctor if any prescription drugs you are taking can raise blood pressure. Birth control pills were first linked to high blood pressure in 1967 by Dr. John Laragh, according to the *Journal of the American Medical Association* (201,918:22). Over the years several other studies have verified the suspicions. The longer "the pill" is used and the older you are when you take it, the higher your chances of developing high blood pressure.

Women taking oral contraceptives should have their blood pressure checked once every two months during the first year. If it is elevated, a different form of birth control should be used. Once "the pill" is stopped, blood pressure should return to a regular level within four months.

There are hundreds of drugs, including over-the-counter diet pills, which list high blood pressure as a side effect. Be sure to read the warnings listed on any non-prescription or prescription drugs you may buy.

Be sure to check with your doctor before discontinuing any medication.

Your sexual habits

One of the questions doctors get asked most by men with high blood pressure is, "Can I still have a regular sex life?" In most cases, patients with high blood pressure can continue their sexual relations with their spouse without any problems. If you do experience unusual symptoms like shortness of breath or chest pain following sex, see your doctor as soon as possible to discuss these problems.

Some drugs prescribed for high blood pressure can cause a reduced sex drive and make it difficult to maintain an erection. However, in a recent study by the University of Connecticut Health Center, Boston University and several other centers, three drugs were compared for their sex-related side effects.

Propranolol and methyldopa were found to cause a decrease in sex drive and made it difficult to maintain an erection, reports a study in the *Archives of Internal Medicine* (148:788-794). Sexual problems were the worst in men over 51 years who were taking methyldopa or propranolol and a diuretic. Captopril, the third drug in the study, did not seem to have any affect on either problem, making it the best choice to avoid sexual problems.

Since doctors believe that some men avoid treatment for high blood pressure because they worry about losing their sex drive, this study is very reassuring.

If you are taking prescription drugs for blood pressure and you think the drugs might be affecting your sex drive, be sure to discuss this with your doctor to see if an alternative drug might work better for you.

Breathing exercises

Daily breathing exercises might help reduce high blood pressure. Practice by lying flat on your back on a carpeted floor. Prop up your head and put a cushion under your knees so you are completely comfortable and relaxed. Breathe in slowly (to the count of 10), hold for two seconds, then breathe out slowly (another count of 10). Many people feel that they are practicing good breathing just by breathing in slowly, but slow exhaling is just as important. By doing these deep breathing exercises for only three to five minutes each day, you will feel relaxed and may lower your blood pressure and pulse rate.

Cancer

Cancer might cause high blood pressure. Several studies have linked high blood pressure and cancer, but a new Canadian study shows that cancer might cause high blood pressure. Until now, many researchers believed that high blood pressure increased one's risk of developing cancer. But, the study in the medical journal *Cancer* (59:7,1386) revealed that blood pressure increased due to the cancer, rather than causing the cancer.

Creatinine

Measuring a common waste product from your body might be the best early warning sign yet discovered to signal your risk of death from high blood pressure.

Researchers have discovered that a blood test frequently performed during routine medical examinations might be a highly accurate predictor of fatality in patients with hypertension.

More than 50 percent of people with a combination of high blood pressure and high levels of a substance called creatinine in the blood will die within eight years, the report says.

Researchers analyzed data from a massive study involving 14 medical schools.

Among the 10,940 high blood pressure patients enrolled in the study, a high level — 2.5 milligrams per deciliter (mg/dl) or more — of a substance called creatinine in their blood serum was associated with a surprisingly high death rate, according to a report in *Hypertension* (13,1:1).

"These data suggest that in patients with high blood pressure and a serum creatinine level equal to or greater than 2.5, more than 50 percent will die within eight years," says Dr. Neil B. Shulman, a principal investigator in the study.

Beginning at a serum creatinine level of 1.2, there was a noticeable continuous increase in risk of death at increasing levels of creatinine, Shulman says.

A normal creatinine range is usually considered to be between 0.7 and 1.5 mg/dl, he adds.

It's not that creatinine by itself causes anything bad to happen.

High levels of it just serve like a smoke detector's buzzer, warning that something bad is going on in the body.

Creatinine is a waste product of metabolic processes in muscle cells, like smoke from a fire, explains Shulman, associate professor of medicine at Emory University in Atlanta.

Normally, the kidneys filter creatinine out of the blood.

For that reason, high levels of creatinine in the blood may indicate kidney problems.

But the patients with high creatinine levels tended to die of heart disease and stroke, not of kidney disease, the scientists found.

"We don't know why the hearts and brains of these patients with kidney dysfunction are so vulnerable to heart attacks and stroke," Shulman says.

The new finding is important, he adds, because it might lead to new approaches to preventing the complications of high blood pressure, which include heart attack and stroke.

According to Shulman, the study indicates that high blood levels of creatinine should be recognized as a risk "marker" for stroke and heart attack.

An abnormal electrocardiogram (ECG) or an enlarged heart are other risk "markers."

Conventional risk factors include cigarette smoking, elevated serum cholesterol and high blood pressure.

"I think our finding will be valuable both to the researchers who are trying to unravel the mysteries of high blood pressure and to the practicing physicians who need to identify which patients deserve special attention," Shulman says.

Patients with high creatinine levels are in such a "risky situation" that physicians should work hard to help them reduce their risk factors for heart attack and stroke, he says.

16

DRUGS AND SIDE EFFECTS

A description of the general types of blood pressure medications

When your doctor prescribes a drug, it belongs to a general category of drugs. All the drugs in the group act in a similar way to solve a problem.

Here are some brief descriptions of the major drug groups used to treat high blood pressure. The drugs are listed with the generic (or chemical name) first, followed by the brand names. Remember that many of the drugs can be purchased in generic form as well as by their brand names.

ACE inhibitors

ACE is an abbreviation of Angiotensin Converting Enzyme. This enzyme converts angiotensin I to angiotensin II, a hormone that causes high blood pressure. ACE inhibitors cause the enzyme to "bind" in the body. When the enzyme is not available, no angiotensin II is produced, and blood pressure is maintained at a regular level. This is a new class of drugs that was introduced in the 1980s.

New research suggests that ACE inhibitors can help your heart just when it needs it the most.

In a recent three-and-a-half-year study of 2,231 heart

attack victims, captopril reduced the risk of a second attack by 25 percent, and cut the risk of developing heart failure by 22 percent. In addition, the risk of death was reduced by 19 percent, reports *The New England Journal of Medicine (327,10:669)*.

A second study involving 4,228 people revealed a 29-percent reduction in the development of heart failure in patients being treated with enalapril, according to the same issue of NEJM. In the people who did develop heart failure, the onset was delayed by 14 months in the group taking enalapril. The drug also reduced hospitalizations by 20 percent. All participants had some damage to the left ventricle, which reduces the heart's pumping efficiency.

A third study, which involved administering enalapril within 24 hours after a heart attack, was stopped after six months because there didn't seem to be any increase in survival rates. The benefits seem to be greater when drugs are given three to 16 days after a heart attack, as in the first study.

Heart attack victims have an increased risk of a second attack because of the damage to the left ventricle. They are also at risk for enlargement of the heart and heart failure, which are major predictors of death. These studies indicate that for some people who already have damaged hearts, ACE inhibitors could be the latest weapons in the fight against heart failure.

ACE inhibitors should be used with caution by people with poor kidney function, autoimmune diseases (like rheumatoid arthritis or lupus), or people on drugs affecting white blood cells or immune response. They should not be used during pregnancy because they can cause injury or even death to the fetus.

While on ACE inhibitor treatment, excessive perspiration, dehydration, vomiting, mouth sores, fever, sore throat, swelling of the hands or feet, irregular heartbeat, chest pains, water retention, skin rash, changes in taste, difficulty in breathing, diarrhea or any signs of infection should be reported to the doctor immediately. Ace inhibitors caused cough in 7 to 25 percent of patients in a recent study reported in the *Archives of Internal Medicine* (152,8:1698). This figure is much higher than previously thought, and researchers suggest physicians try prescribing smaller doses. Over-the-counter cough, cold or allergy medications should be avoided. Aspirin or indomethacin decreases the effectiveness of captopril and should be avoided. Patients also taking diuretics may experience severe loss of blood pressure during the first three hours after receiving the first dose of an ACE inhibitor. ACE inhibitors most frequently prescribed are:

- benazepril (Lotensin)
- captopril (Capoten)
- enalapril (Vasotec)
- fosinopril (Monopril)
- lisinopril (Prinivil, Zestril)
- ramipril (Altace)

Beta blockers

Your body has a type of built-in alarm system that switches on whenever you face an emergency or any sort of stressful situation. This is called the emergency nervous system, and it causes you to put forth your best efforts to deal with stressful situations.

If your blood pressure is normal, your alarm system is probably functioning as it is meant to — now and then raising your energy level, your "get up and go," and making you a capable, productive person.

If your blood pressure is high, however, your alarm system may be turned on too much of the time. You may not feel tense, but your nervous system could be too active. This could be an inherited condition, or it could result from your life situation.

Beta-adrenergic blocking agents, known as beta blockers, work to keep your emergency nervous system blocked so that your heart will beat more slowly and your blood pressure will fall. They block the action of naturally occurring substances, like epinephrine (adrenaline), that stimulate the heart. These substances, which are released into the circulation in response to physical exertion or other stress, cause an increase in heart rate and in the force with which the heart pumps blood. By decreasing the rate and force of the heart contraction, beta blockers reduce blood pressure levels. They are also used to treat angina and abnormal heart rhythms and can be used in the treatment of atrial fibrillation. Some beta blockers are used to treat heart attack victims because they seem to be beneficial in lowering the rate of having a second heart attack in certain patients.

Unfortunately, these drugs may also cause depression and dull your energy levels, leaving you drowsy or feeling lethargic most of the time. You may begin to feel like you don't care much about life anymore and chalk it up to just "getting older." Often these feelings come on so gradually that you may not realize that it is the drug that is causing you to feel this way.

There is evidence that chromium, a trace element, helps counteract beta blockers bad effects on cholesterol. Beta blockers are often used to treat hypertension in older people. But, they lower HDL levels to such a degree that the risk of coronary heart disease may not be decreased. In a study reported in *Annals of Internal Medicine* (115,12:917-924), researchers found that 600 micrograms of chromium per day significantly raised HDL, and reduced the risk of coronary heart disease by 12 to 17 percent in men who took beta blockers three times a day.

Beta blockers should not be used (or be used with great caution) by people with asthma, hay fever, a history of congestive heart failure and in pregnancy. Beta blockers may interfere with heart activity during major surgery and with the treatment of overactive thyroid, low blood sugar, diabetes, kidney disease or liver disease. Beta blockers may change the effectiveness of insulin, anti-inflammatory drugs, antihistamines and antidiabetic drugs. Avoid alcohol. Alcohol can cause dangerously low blood pressure when combined with a beta blocker. Smoking may reduce the effectiveness of the beta blocker propranolol.

If you have been taking a beta blocker and suddenly stop, your body may react by raising your blood pressure to dangerously high rates. If you want to stop taking medication, you must do it gradually and under the watchful care and consent of your doctor. Beta blockers most frequently prescribed include:

- acebutolol (Sectral)
- atenolol (Tenormin)
- betaxolol (Kerlone)
- carteolol (Cartrol)
- labetalol (Normodyne, Trandate)
- metoprolol (Lopressor)
- nadolol (Corgard)
- penbutolol (Levatol)
- pindolol (Visken)
- propranolol (Inderal, Inderal LA)
- timolol (Blocadren)

Vasodilators

These drugs act on the muscles of the blood vessels causing them to dilate and so lowering blood pressure. Side effects can include headache, flushing, stuffy nose, stomach upsets and rapid heart rate. Hydralazine may produce symptoms of rheumatoid arthritis or acute lupus erythematosus (like rheumatoid arthritis with skin rashes) when used over a long period of time, or by people who are slow to break down the drug. Minoxidil is usually used in more severe cases, and sodium nitroprusside is usually reserved for hypertensive emergencies.

- hydralazine (Alazine, Apresoline)
- minoxidil (Loniten, Minodyl)
- sodium nitroprusside (Nipride, Nitropress)

Antiadrenergic agents

Centrally acting drugs

Drugs in this group act on the sympathetic nervous system which controls involuntary responses to stressful situations. They can cause drowsiness, depression, excessive dreaming, diarrhea and nausea.

According to a report in *Medical World News* (31,6:11), clonidine can slow down a patient's recovery after a stroke. Dr. Larry B. Goldstein and his colleagues at Duke University Medical Center studied records of 58 stroke patients to determine the effects of different drugs on recovery. Of the 58 patients, 24 took clonidine at the time of their stroke or during their treatment. Patients who did not take clonidine improved more quickly than those who did.

- clonidine (Catapres)
- guanabenz (Wytensin)
- guanfacine (Tenex)

- methyldopa (Aldomet, Amodopa)

Peripherally acting drugs

These drugs act in various ways on the sympathetic nerve endings to dilate blood vessels and are used to treat severe hypertension. Guanethidine-type drugs can cause low blood pressure and a loss of balance when you stand quickly. Drinking alcohol, exercising or hot weather can aggravate this side effect. Diarrhea, fluid retention, stuffy nose, dry mouth and sexual problems in men are also common. People with a history of depression should not take reserpine, since it can cause severe depression even in someone without depression problems in the past. Drugs in this group include:

- deserpidine (Harmonyl)
- doxazosin (Cardura)
- guanadrel (Hylorel)
- guanethidine (Ismelin Sulfate)
- prazosin (Minipress)
- rescinnamine (Moderil)
- reserpine (Serpalan, Serpasil)
- terazosin (Hytrin)

Calcium channel blockers

These medicines interfere with the transport of calcium into the heart and vein muscle cells and inhibit their contraction. This causes the veins and arteries to enlarge and reduce the heart rate and blood pressure. Calcium channel blockers are mostly used to treat angina. However, some calcium channel blockers can also be used in the management of high blood pressure.

Dizziness, light-headedness, flushing and fluid retention are just some of the side effects of this class of drugs.

Calcium channel blockers lower the hypertensive's risk of coronary artery disease suggests Dr. James Sowers in *Postgraduate Medicine* (92,2:265). Dr. Sowers is professor of medicine and physiology and director of endocrinology and hypertension division at Wayne State University School of Medicine. Most antihypertensive drugs do not sufficiently lower the risk of coronary artery disease because of their affect on cholesterol and other blood fats. In human and animal studies, some calcium channel blockers have been found to inhibit the development of atherosclerosis.

Physicians are decreasing their use of calcium channel blockers after a heart attack, according to *The New England Journal of Medicine* (327,4:242). Results of a study of diltiazem that was also reported in *The New England Journal of Medicine* (319,7:385) showed the drug can help lower the rates of second heart attack and death in some people. However, for many patients, particularly those with pulmonary (lung) congestion, diltiazem can increase the risks.

But calcium channel blockers can help protect your kidneys, say researchers in the *Archives of Internal Medicine* (152,8:1573). These drugs can open up constricted veins, cause the kidneys to flush out sodium faster and protect against kidney failure. They are even thought to protect transplanted kidneys against damage. People with high blood pressure seem to be more sensitive to the beneficial effects of calcium channel blockers than people with normal blood pressure levels. This is all good news for people with kidney-problem-induced high blood pressure.

Taking beta blockers at the same time as calcium channel blockers is usually well tolerated, but they may cause heart failure in people with aorta problems who are also taking beta blockers. Don't withdraw suddenly from beta blockers before or during calcium-channel-blocker therapy. Some calcium channel blockers should be used with caution in patients with congestive heart failure. Prescriptions for calcium-channel blockers include:

- diltiazem (Cardizem, Cardizem SR, Cardizem CD)
- felodipine (Plendil)
- isradipine (DynaCirc)
- nicardipine (Cardene, Cardene SR)
- nifedipine (Procardia XL)
- verapamil (Calan, Calan SR, Isoptin, Isoptin SR, Verelan)

Diuretics

Diuretics are probably the most commonly recommended high blood pressure drugs, with thiazides comprising the largest group in this class.

Often called "water pills," diuretics are chemicals which act on the kidneys, causing them to flush salt and water from the body. To understand how these drugs lower blood pressure, you must remember how important our kidneys are to our health. One of the main jobs of our kidneys is to flush out excess salt and minerals from our bodies each day. However, if over the years we've eaten too much salt or are salt retentive, the kidneys can't take salt out fast enough, and it builds up in our bodies. We then retain extra fluid to dilute the salt.

Our bodies begin to sense a problem — there's too much salt and fluid building up in the system. So, to solve the problem our blood pressure rises, forcing the kidneys to flush out the extra salt and fluids.

The function of the diuretics is to help the kidney take out the excess salt and fluid so that our blood pressure doesn't have to rise to do the job. As fluid volume in the blood vessels drops, the blood pressure also goes down.

Diuretics are also prescribed to add to the effectiveness of other blood-pressure-reducing drugs.

One problem with this type of drug is that it may be hard to find one that will really work well in your particular body. Either they simply aren't sufficient or they are too potent and make you run to the bathroom continually. To find the right drug at the right dose for you can be very difficult.

Also, if you continue to eat a lot of salt and you are on a diuretic that is flushing it out of your system, the drug will also be flushing out too many other minerals from your body, like potassium. It has been estimated that the majority of patients receiving diuretics exhibit one or more of the signs and symptoms of low potassium. Therefore, potassium supplements are usually prescribed as well, unless the patient is receiving "potassium sparing" diuretics.

Thiazide diuretics should be used with caution by people with poor kidney function or progressive liver disease. Sensitivity reactions are most likely to occur in people with allergies or bronchial asthma. Thiazide diuretics can cause severe sunburn with modest exposure to the sun. Insulin requirements may have to be adjusted. Pain relievers and barbiturates may cause increased effects of the diuretics and should be avoided if possible. Thiazide diuretics also interact with digitalis and related drugs, adrenocorticoids and tricyclic antidepressant drugs.

Loop diurectics are so called because they also work in the loop of Henle, a specific part of the kidney, which helps make them much more effective. Dosages should be individualized and carefully monitored.

Clearly, the diuretic drugs, though they are very often prescribed, are not without serious drawbacks. One recent study showed that patients with unstable angina who received thiazide diuretics had higher death rates than those who didn't. Commonly prescribed diuretic drugs include:

Thiazide and similar diuretics

- bendroflumethiazide (Naturetin)
- benzthiazide (Aquatag, Exna, Hydrex, Marazide, Proaqua)
- chlorothiazide (Diachlor, Diurigen, Diuril)

- chlorthalidone (Hygroton, Hylidone, Thalitone)
- cyclothiazide (Anhydron)
- hydrochlorothiazide (Diaqua, Esidrix, Hydro-Chlor, HydroDIURIL, Hydromal, Hydro-T, Hydro-Z-50, Hydrozide-50, Mictrin, Oretic, Thiuretic)
- hydroflumethiazide (Diucardin, Saluron)
- indapamide (Lozol)
- methyclothiazide (Aquatensen, Enduron, Ethon)
- metolazone (Diulo, Mykrox, Zaroxolyn)
- polythiazide (Renese)
- quinethazone (Hydromox)
- trichlormethiazide (Diurese, Metahydrin, Naqua, Niazide, Trichlorex)

Loop diuretics

- bumetanide (Bumex)
- ethacrynic acid (Edecrin)
- furosemide (Fumide, Lasix, Luramide)

Potassium-sparing diuretics

- amiloride (Midamor)
- spironolactone (Alatone, Aldactone)
- triamterene (Dyrenium)

Combinations

Combinations of different types of drugs are sometimes used to make it easier for people to remember to take their medication and to have the most efficient use of the drugs in the body. They are not usually given as the initial treatment for high blood pressure, since the individual doses of each drug need to be adjusted separately before the optimum combination for each person can be obtained. Here are some combinations that are often prescribed:

Diuretic combinations

- amiloride and hydrochlorothiazide (Moduretic)
- spironolactone and hydrochlorothiazide (Alazide, Aldactazide, Spironazide, Spirozide)
- triamterene and hydrochlorothiazide (Dyazide, Maxzide)

Antihypertensive combinations

- bendroflumethiazide and nadolol (Corzide)
- chlorothiazide and methyldopa (Aldoclor)
- chlorothiazide and reserpine (Chloroserpine, Diupres)
- chlorthalidone and atenolol (Tenoretic)
- chlorthalidone and clonidine (Combipres)
- chlorthalidone and reserpine (Demi-Regroton, Regroton)
- hydrochlorothiazide and deserpidine (Oreticyl)
- hydrochlorothiazide and hydralazine (Apresazide, Apresoline-Esidrix, Aprozide, Hydra-Zide)
- hydrochlorothiazide, hydralazine and reserpine (Cam-ap-es, H-H-R, Ser-A-Gen, Seralazide, Ser-Ap-Es, Serpazide, Tri-Hydroserpine, Unipres)

- hydrochlorothiazide and reserpine (Hydropres, Hydro-Serp, Hydroserpine, Hydrosine, Mallopress, Serpasil-Esidrix)
- hydrochlorothiazide and captopril (Capozide)
- hydrochlorothiazide and enalapril (Vaseretic)
- hydrochlorothiazide and guanethidine monosulfate (Esimil)
- hydrochlorothiazide and labetalol (Normozide, Trandate HCT)
- hydrochlorothiazide and methyldopa (Aldoril, Alodopa)
- hydrochlorothiazide and metoprolol (Lopressor HCT)
- hydrochlorothiazide and propranolol HCI (Inderide, Inderide LA)
- hydrochlorothiazide and timolol maleate (Timolide)
- hydroflumethiazide and reserpine (Hydropine, Salazide, Salazide-Demi, Salutensin, Salutensin-Demi)
- methychlothiazide and deserpidine (Enduronyl)
- methychlothiazide and reserpine (Diutensen-R)
- polythiazide and prazosin (Minizide)
- polythiazide and reserpine (Renese-R)
- quinethazone and reserpine (Hydromox R)
- trichlormethiazide and reserpine (Diurese-R, Metatensin, Naquival)

MAO inhibitors

Another group of drugs that works by inhibiting a normal

body action is the monoamine oxidase (MAO) inhibitors. They stop the body from producing certain chemicals in the brain and nerves.

MAO inhibitors are antidepressant drugs and have many side effects like dizziness and weakness. Lowering blood pressure is really just one more side effect. For that reason some MAO inhibitors have been used in the past to treat high blood pressure. MAO inhibiting drugs can also have more serious side effects. We have not listed the drugs as they are not normally used in the treatment of high blood pressure, but people using these drugs should exercise caution because of the effects they can have on blood pressure.

Potassium supplements

Potassium is a mineral that is needed to offset the side effects of certain blood pressure reducing drugs which lower the body's potassium to below normal levels. And a low potassium level is itself a risk factor for high blood pressure. Potassium supplements are often needed as it would not be practical to eat enough potassium-rich foods to compensate for the loss, according to a report in *The New England Journal of Medicine* (313:582-582).

Tablet forms of potassium salts can cause stomach irritation or even ulcers in some people, so liquid forms are usually safest. Forms of potassium available include:
- potassium bicarbonate (K+Care ET)
- potassium chloride (Cena-K, Kaochlor, Kay Ciel, Klorvess, Potasalan, Rum-K)

- potassium gluconate (Kaon, Kaylixir, K-G Elixir)
- potassium combinations (Effer-K, Kolyum, Klor-Con/EF, K-Lyte, K-Lyte DS, Tri-K, Twin-K

The effectiveness of prescription drugs

The only truly safe way to help lower your blood pressure is to stop doing what's causing it if you can. If you have practiced all the natural ways we have discussed, and your doctor still feels you need medication, be sure you know and monitor the drug or drugs you are taking so that you can advise your doctor of any side effects. Also, you can help him determine whether any drug is actually doing what it was intended to do.

17

IF DRUGS ARE PRESCRIBED

Prescription drugs and lowering blood pressure naturally

You've now read all about high blood pressure and how it can be lowered naturally. You've also read about the types of medicine you may be taking. Where does this leave you? This chapter will help you decide how best to handle your blood pressure problem.

When is blood pressure medication prescribed?

Drug treatment for mild to moderate high blood pressure has been extremely controversial within the medical profession because physicians are not sure when blood pressure levels are high enough to begin using prescription drugs. A study in Sweden found that reducing blood pressure to lower than 150/85 in middle-age men had no effect on their risk of heart or artery disease. The study at the University of Goteberg was conducted over 12 years, according to the *Journal of the American Medical Association* (259:2553).

However, another new study has shown that early drug treatment can save lives. People with mild high blood pressure who took drugs had 40 percent fewer fatal strokes and 38 percent fewer non-fatal strokes, in research that Dr. Charles Hennekens presented to an American Heart Association meeting in San Francisco. Therefore, treating mild or moderate high blood pressure with drugs might save lives. There continues to be a lot of controversy on the best use of drugs in people with low or moderate hypertension.

In spite of the controversy, high blood pressure is usually treated with drugs. Most people with high blood pressure need drug treatment, according to a study by the Joint National Committee on Detection, Evaluation, and Treatment of High Blood Pressure, reported the *Archives of Internal Medicine* (144:1045).

Prescription drugs can have positive benefits. They are the most common treatment because they are easy to prescribe and easy for the patient to take.

Prescription drugs are often overprescribed because many physicians are reluctant to offer any alternatives to drugs to their patients. It is difficult for a doctor to make sure that his patient takes the prescribed medicine. It would be impossible for him to ensure that a diet and exercise plan was being followed. Most people want "a pill" from the doctor that will magically make them better.

If high blood pressure is diagnosed, your doctor should review your family history and administer some tests to make sure that it hasn't affected any of your vital organs. Your doctor should also test for rare causes of high blood pressure, like kidney problems, Cushing's disease or brain tumors.

A new procedure, involving resting for half an hour, taking the drug captopril and then having a special blood test will help doctors determine if narrow kidney arteries are causing your blood pressure problems. Narrow arteries leading to one or both kidneys causes high blood pressure in just one to five percent of all high blood pressure cases. If it's discovered, your doctor might decide you need angioplasty, a technique used to widen narrowed arteries using a balloon catheter.

Blood pressure was reduced in 90 percent of over 200 patients who had narrow kidney arteries and were treated by angioplasty, Dr. Heinrich Ingrisch reported from the Bogenhausen Clinic in Munich. The success continued as 75 percent had normal blood pressure six months after the angioplasty, and of those, 77 percent maintained normal levels five years after surgery.

Yet, if high blood pressure from kidney-artery malfunctions goes undiagnosed, a person may be needlessly treated for high blood pressure.

Your eyes, stomach, blood vessels in the legs, kidney function, heart and nervous system should be checked. A complete blood count including thyroid hormone and renin levels, urinalysis (an analysis of the urine), a chest X-ray, and an electrocardiogram (ECG) may also be needed to determine the damage, if any, to your heart, arteries and kidneys. Insulin levels should also be checked.

High levels of thyroid hormone in the blood may show

that an overactive thyroid is causing or aggravating the high blood pressure. High or low levels of renin, a substance produced by the kidneys, can also affect the preferred treatment.

All of these factors will help determine whether or not your doctor will prescribe blood pressure medicine and, if needed, what kind of drug will be best for you.

Drug treatment is quite complex because many people have more than one ailment and need several different drugs. The interaction of those drugs and the actions that the drugs have on the body have to be considered for each person. For example, some people with high blood pressure may also have heart problems or high cholesterol levels which will need to be considered when deciding on the correct medication for that person.

Drugs of first choice

Since many factors enter into blood pressure control, many different drugs are used for treatment. Usually doctors try the most widely accepted drugs first — drugs that usually work best for most people. However, if these drugs don't control the blood pressure, other drugs that are stronger, more expensive or have more serious side effects are tried.

Diuretic drugs are usually prescribed first because they are effective in many people and are relatively inexpensive. ACE inhibitors and calcium channel blockers can also be used as the first step in drug treatment, but these drugs are much more expensive.

Medical Letter consultants suggest that "if a diuretic is not chosen as the initial drug and a second drug is necessary, then a diuretic should be used."

Considering the cost factor

Of an estimated 60 million Americans with high blood pressure, about 19 million are currently being treated with available medications. If they only take one kind (and many people need combinations), twice a day, that comes to 38 million tablets swallowed daily. Medication alone costs billions of dollars each year. On top of that, consider the cost of work time lost by the patients and the doctors' time.

What should you know if you are taking medication?

Here are some tips for people taking medicine to control high blood pressure:

• Get your blood pressure checked regularly. It only takes a minute or two.

• Take your prescribed medicine as directed. Keep doing so because, even if you feel better, your high blood pressure is not cured. Regular dosages are necessary to keep it under control.

• Don't change the dose yourself. You might get too much or too little medicine. Either way it could be harmful. If you take less of your prescription than your doctor prescribes, you may increase the risk of complications such as stroke or heart attack. If you take more of your medication than you're supposed to, you increase the risk of having side effects from the drug.

• Don't stop taking a drug on your own, even if you feel light-headed, dizzy, tired, depressed or have trouble sleeping. Your drug can be controlling your blood pressure but might also be giving you these or other side effects. Notify your doctor immediately when bothersome side effects occur. Many times your doctor will be able to give you a different drug. Your doctor needs to know how medication is affecting you in order to treat your condition properly.

• If you have questions about your high blood pressure or your prescription, don't ask a friend or relative. Their information or advice may be well-intended but wrong for you. Ask your doctor or pharmacist — they are the people qualified to answer your questions.

• Be sure to tell your doctor and pharmacist about all prescription drugs, any daily vitamin or mineral supplements, or non-prescription drugs (aspirin, cold medicines, laxatives) that you take regularly. Many drugs interact with each other and lose or gain potency or cause serious side effects when taken together.

• Get all your prescriptions filled at the same pharmacy. This will help you keep track of them.

• Record any side effects you may experience while taking prescription drugs, and report them to your doctor.

• Always follow label instructions. If there is a difference between your doctor's verbal instructions and the label instructions, contact your doctor immediately. If you don't follow the doctor's specific instructions, your medicine may be ineffective or harmful to you.

• Never take drugs prescribed for someone else. Drugs should be prescribed after considering other drugs being taken, one's age, weight, health history and other important factors. Exchanging medicine is dangerous. Don't do it!

• Ask questions about the drugs your doctor prescribes. If you learn more about your prescriptions, you can understand why you should take your drugs properly so they will be most effective. If you are well-informed about your treatment and condition, you will know if something unusual occurs, and you will know when to contact your doctor for help. Do not be afraid to write down your doctor's answers to these questions so you can refer to them later.

- What is the name of the drug?
- What is it supposed to do?
- How long will it take before it is effective?
- How am I supposed to take it?
- When am I supposed to take it?
- Are there any foods, drinks, other drugs or activities that I should avoid while taking this drug?
- What are the drug's side effects?
- What should I do if the side effects happen to me?
- Is written information available on this drug that I could have?
- How can I get this written information?

• Keep a list of all your current prescriptions in your wallet or purse. Include the name of the drug and what dose you are taking. When you visit your doctor, have him check your list and keep it up to date. The list will remind him of your current prescriptions, and keeping it with you could help avoid dangerous drug interactions. During an emergency, the list will provide valuable information for the attending doctor.

• Ibuprofen, an over-the-counter pain reliever, may interfere with prescription drugs controlling blood pressure, according to research by the University of Cincinnati Medical Center (*Annals of Internal Medicine*). Blood pressure levels increased about seven points in just three weeks in patients who took ibuprofen for pain while receiving blood pressure medicine. Increased blood pressure did not occur when aspirin or acetaminophen was used for pain, the study reports.

Ibuprofen is found in many prescription and over-the-counter medicines for pain (usually arthritis or menstrual pain) including Advil, Excedrin IB, Haltran, Ibuprin, Medipren, Midol, Motrin IB, Nuprin, Pamprin-IB and Trendar. The doctors in the study suggest that patients taking any type of blood pressure medicine should refrain from using ibuprofen.

• Even if you are taking a prescription drug with your doctor's knowledge, you should still try to eat foods low in salt, improve your diet, get regular exercise and do all the things you can to help lower your blood pressure naturally. These changes will enable your doctor to prescribe the least amount of medication possible. In one study at the Indiana

University School of Medicine, one-third of people who cut back on sodium were able to reduce their blood pressure and their medication (*Journal of the American Medical Association* 259:2561).

What are the disadvantages of blood pressure medications?

Long-term treatment with blood pressure reducing drugs may increase the chance of developing diabetes in middle-age men, reports a study in the *British Medical Journal* (298,6681:1147). But the risk seems to be greater in men who are "predisposed" to diabetes, according to Dr. Einar T. Skarfos who lead the Swedish study. The study does not prove that blood pressure drugs cause some cases of diabetes, but it suggests that continued use may trigger the disease in some cases.

Blood pressure drugs can cause miserable side effects like headaches, poor appetite, upset stomach, dry mouth, diarrhea, stuffy nose, tingling or numbness in hands or feet, dizziness, cramps, depression, rashes, chills, fever, constipation, aching joints, difficult urination or low sex drive.

A study reported in the *Journal of the American Medical Association* (253:3263) involving 3,844 patients with high blood pressure found that 9.3 percent of them stopped drug treatment because of "definite" or "probable" side effects, and an additional 23.4 percent stopped drug treatment because of "possible" side effects.

Drug treatment is only effective when the drugs are

taken as prescribed. Since high blood pressure may not have symptoms, many people stop taking their medication because they feel better. Other people forget to take their prescriptions. This can lead to dangerously high blood pressure levels. Never stop taking or change anything about your prescribed medication without your doctor's knowledge and consent.

Remember that high blood pressure is not "cured," but it can be controlled. Learning to control your blood pressure is a lifelong commitment. If you and your doctor choose non-drug methods, they must be continued for the rest of your life, just as prescription drugs would be.

Choosing just one area, like reducing salt intake, may or may not help lower your blood pressure. But it is the effective combination of natural methods that will give you the best results. For example, many people try exercising or eating a low-sodium, high-potassium diet. In a study by Dr. James Mitchell in *Psychosomatic Medicine*, people lowered their diastolic pressure about 10 points by dieting or exercising. But when they combined diet and exercise, they lowered their blood pressure an additional four points.

The first step you should take to lower your blood pressure naturally is to talk with your doctor about the methods we've described. Have your doctor monitor your blood pressure levels as you gradually make changes in your diet and lifestyle. Your doctor will probably be as excited as you are when your body gradually needs less and less of the medication.

18

FOURTEEN-DAY MENUS

Daily menus

The menus that follow recommend foods that are high in fiber and low in cholesterol, fat, salt and calories. Check with your doctor before you use this plan. The foods that are underlined are included in the recipe section. To add extra flavor, try these tips:

- Spread one teaspoon of jam, marmalade or honey (never butter) on toast or muffins.
- Add a little mustard and lots of lettuce to your sandwiches.
- Top baked potatoes with cottage cheese, light cream cheese, spring onions or a little low-fat margarine.
- To make vegetables more interesting, flavor with lemon juice, mint, parsley or freshly ground pepper.
- If you must sauté, do so in a little olive oil.

First day

Breakfast: 1 cup oatmeal made with skim milk,
sweetened with bananas or raisins
1 small glass unsweetened orange juice
1 piece whole wheat toast
Water, decaffeinated coffee, tea or
skim milk

Lunch: Sliced chicken sandwich on whole wheat bread
Lettuce, tomato and bean salad (make your own
oil-free dressing with vinegar, water and seasonings)
1 cup fresh fruit salad
Water

Dinner: 4 oz broiled veal
1 piece <u>bran</u> <u>bread</u>
1 cup green beans
3/4 cup <u>brown</u> <u>rice</u>
Green salad
Water, decaffeinated coffee or tea

Second day

Breakfast: 2 pieces cinnamon toast (use whole wheat or
homemade <u>bran</u> <u>bread</u>)
1 glass unsweetened orange juice
Water, decaffeinated coffee or tea

Lunch: 1 <u>tuna</u> <u>salad</u> sandwich on whole wheat or <u>bran</u>
<u>bread</u>
1 unpeeled apple
Skim milk

Dinner: 1 <u>bran</u> <u>muffin</u>
1 serving <u>cod</u> <u>and</u> <u>rice</u> <u>bake</u>
1 cup lima beans

1 peach
Water, decaffeinated coffee or tea

Third day

Breakfast: 2 slices whole wheat or homemade <u>bran</u> <u>bread</u>
1/2 grapefruit, unsweetened
Water, decaffeinated coffee, tea or skim milk

Lunch: 1 serving <u>cottage</u> <u>cheese</u> <u>and</u> <u>cucumber</u> <u>salad</u>
1 apple or peach
Water

Dinner: 4 oz <u>meat</u> <u>loaf</u>
1 baked potato
1 cup stewed tomatoes
1 <u>dinner</u> <u>roll</u>
Water, decaffeinated coffee or tea

Fourth day

Breakfast: 2 <u>bran</u> <u>muffins</u>
1 glass unsweetened orange juice
Water, decaffeinated coffee or tea

Lunch: Sliced turkey sandwich on whole wheat
or <u>bran</u> <u>bread</u>
1 raw carrot
Skim milk

Dinner: 4 oz broiled ground beef patty
1 serving <u>kidney</u> <u>bean</u> or <u>three</u>-<u>bean</u> <u>salad</u>
1 <u>dinner</u> <u>roll</u>
1 cup tomato soup (low sodium)
1 <u>brownie</u>
Water, decaffeinated coffee or tea

Fifth day

Breakfast: 1 carton low-fat yogurt
1 piece whole wheat or <u>bran</u> <u>bread</u> toast
1/2 cup prunes
Water, decaffeinated coffee or tea

Lunch: 6 oz <u>tuna</u> <u>salad</u>
1 dinner roll
1/2 cup <u>easy</u>-<u>cooked</u> <u>beets</u>
1 <u>brownie</u>
Water

Dinner: Grilled cheese sandwich on whole wheat or <u>bran</u> <u>bread</u>
(Use 1oz of low-fat cheese and grill without butter in a non-stick pan.)
1 cup vegetable soup
Water, decaffeinated coffee or tea

Sixth day

Breakfast: 1 bowl oatmeal

1 glass unsweetened fruit juice
Water, decaffeinated coffee, or tea

Lunch: 1 cup <u>brown</u> <u>rice</u> salad
1 cup fresh fruit
1 <u>dinner</u> <u>roll</u>
Water

Dinner: 1 cup <u>macaroni</u> <u>and</u> <u>cheese</u>
1 cup green beans
1 <u>dinner</u> <u>roll</u>
Water, decaffeinated coffee, tea or skim milk

Seventh day

Breakfast: 1 bowl oatmeal with banana
1 glass unsweetened pineapple juice
Water, decaffeinated coffee or tea

Lunch: 1 <u>tuna</u> <u>salad</u> sandwich on whole wheat
or <u>bran</u> <u>bread</u>
1 cup fresh fruit
Skim milk

Dinner: 4 oz roast beef
4 new potatoes, boiled in skins
1 <u>dinner</u> <u>roll</u>
1/2 cup carrots
1 <u>brownie</u>
Water, decaffeinated coffee or tea

Eighth day

Breakfast: 1 bowl whole-grain cereal with 1 cup unsweetened strawberries
Water, decaffeinated coffee, tea or skim milk

Lunch: Grilled cheese sandwich on whole wheat or <u>bran</u> <u>bread</u> (see *Fifth Day*)
1 cup vegetable soup
Water

Dinner: 4 oz broiled veal
1/2 cup peas
1 cup broccoli
2 slices whole wheat or <u>bran</u> <u>bread</u>
Water, decaffeinated coffee or tea

Ninth day

Breakfast: 1 bowl whole-grain cereal with skim milk
1 orange or 1/2 grapefruit, unsweetened
Water, decaffeinated coffee or tea

Lunch: 1 cup field peas
1 cup stewed tomatoes
Whole-grain crackers (check label to make sure that crackers are low in fat, salt and sugar)
Skim milk

Dinner: 1 piece baked chicken (moisten in skim milk, dip in bread crumbs and bake)
1 baked potato
1 cup steamed carrots
Water, decaffeinated coffee or tea

Tenth day

Breakfast: 1 bowl oatmeal with sliced bananas and skim milk
1 piece whole wheat toast or bran bread
Water, decaffeinated coffee or tea

Lunch: 3/4 cup macaroni and cheese
Green salad
Water

Dinner: 1 lean lamb chop
1 cup spinach
1 baked potato
1 dinner roll
1 peach
Water, decaffeinated coffee or tea

Eleventh day

Breakfast: 1 bowl whole-grain cereal with 1 cup unsweetened strawberries
1 piece whole wheat toast or bran bread
Water, decaffeinated coffee or tea

Lunch: 1 large slice pita bread
1 cup bean soup
Skim milk

Dinner: 4 oz broiled fish
1 cup new potatoes
1 cup asparagus
1 dinner roll
Water, decaffeinated coffee or tea

Twelfth day

Breakfast: 1 bran muffin
1/2 grapefruit, unsweetened
Water, decaffeinated coffee or tea

Lunch: Tuna salad sandwich on whole wheat or bran bread
1/2 cup rice pudding
1 unpeeled apple
Water

Dinner: 1 cup macaroni and cheese
1 cup green beans
1 dinner roll
Water, decaffeinated coffee or tea

Thirteenth day

Breakfast: 1 bowl oatmeal, sweetened with bananas or

raisins
1 <u>bran</u> <u>muffin</u>
1 glass unsweetened orange juice
Water, decaffeinated coffee or tea

Lunch: Sliced chicken sandwich on whole wheat
or <u>bran</u> <u>bread</u>
1 cup <u>kidney</u> <u>bean</u> <u>salad</u>
1 peach
Skim milk

Dinner: 1 serving <u>cod</u> <u>and</u> <u>rice</u> <u>bake</u>
1/2 cup <u>easy-cooked</u> <u>beets</u>
1 piece whole wheat or <u>bran</u> <u>bread</u>
1 <u>brownie</u>
Water, decaffeinated coffee or tea

Fourteenth day

Breakfast: 2 pieces cinnamon toast on whole wheat or <u>bran</u>
<u>bread</u>
1 glass unsweetened orange juice
Water, decaffeinated coffee or tea

Lunch: Grilled cheese sandwich on whole wheat or
<u>bran</u> <u>bread</u> (see *Fifth Day*)
1 cup vegetable soup
1 <u>brownie</u>
Water

Dinner: 4 oz <u>meat</u> <u>loaf</u>
1 baked potato
1 cup broccoli
1 unpeeled apple
Water, decaffeinated coffee, tea or skim milk

19

HEALTHFUL RECIPES

BEAN CROQUETTES

2 cups red kidney beans, cooked
1 cup split peas, cooked
1 cup lentils, cooked
1/4 cup soy grits
1/2 cup homemade chicken stock
1/4 teaspoon freshly ground black pepper
2 egg whites, beaten
2 tablespoons skim milk
1 cup whole wheat bread crumbs, seasoned

Mix beans, peas and lentils and then puree. Combine with grits and seasoning. Add chicken stock. Shape into croquettes. Combine beaten egg whites and skim milk. Dip croquettes in the egg mixture and roll in seasoned bread crumbs. Place under broiler, turning until all sides are brown. Serve hot.

BEANS WITH ONIONS

1/2 lb. dried kidney beans
2 ripe tomatoes, quartered
1 medium onion, chopped
1 medium bell pepper, chopped
chili powder to taste

Soak beans in water overnight, then follow cooking instructions on the package, eliminating salt. Add tomatoes, onion, bell pepper and chili powder. Simmer for an additional 1 to 2 hours or until beans are done.

BEANS, REFRIED

1/2 lb. dried kidney or pinto beans
3/4 cup onion, chopped
3 cloves garlic, crushed
oregano
freshly ground black pepper

Follow cooking instructions on the package, except leave out the salt. Add chopped onion and garlic before simmering. When beans are done (they should be soft and split), drain and season lightly with oregano and pepper. Mash the beans and cook over medium heat in a non-stick skillet until beans begin to dry out. Serve hot.

BEEF STEW

2 onions, chopped
2 lbs. extra lean stew meat
water
5 carrots, diced
4 medium-size potatoes, cubed (leave the skins on)
1 cup corn

Brown the meat and onions in a non-stick skillet over medium heat. Add just enough water to cover meat and vegetables and simmer for 2 hours. Add the remaining ingredients and simmer for another hour.

BEET AND CUCUMBER SALAD, TOSSED

8 to 10 large lettuce leaves
1 large cooked beet
1/2 large cucumber

Tear lettuce leaves into small pieces. Wash cucumber well and dice, unpeeled. Dice beet and toss with cucumber and lettuce.

BEETS, EASY-COOKED

1 lb. beets, thinly sliced
1 teaspoon lemon juice
2 1/2 tablespoons water

Place beets, lemon juice and water in a non-stick skillet. Cover and cook over medium heat, stirring frequently, until tender. Serve hot.

BRAN BREAD AND DINNER ROLLS

1/2 cup warm water
1/4 cup vegetable oil
2 packages active dry yeast
2 1/2 cups skim milk
1/4 cup honey
7 cups stone-ground whole wheat flour, mixed
with 2 cups white flour
1 cup unprocessed bran (see Note)

Let yeast stand in slightly warm, but not hot, water for 5 minutes. Boil milk and then add honey. Cool for 15 minutes and place in large mixing bowl with oil, yeast and 2 cups of flour. Mix thoroughly and add bran. Add rest of flour gradually as you knead the dough. If dough is still sticky, knead in more flour. Place dough in a bowl and let rise for 1 hour and 45 minutes. Then put in 3 or 4 non-stick loaf pans or roll pans. Let rise again for 1 hour. Bake loaves for about 40 minutes at 350°. Bake rolls for 10 minutes at 425°.

Note: Pure, unprocessed bran is different from 100% bran cereal. You can use either type in these recipes, but the texture will be slightly different.

Bran Muffins

3 cups whole wheat flour
2 cups pure unprocessed bran
3 tablespoons honey
1 1/2 packages active dry yeast
2 1/4 cups skim milk
1/2 cup dark molasses
1 egg white
1/2 cup warm water

Heat milk until scalding, then add honey and molasses. Let the milk mixture cool for at least 15 minutes, then add the bran. Add yeast to warm water and set aside for 5 minutes. Add yeast and wheat flour to bran mixture. Beat the egg white and fold into batter. Let stand in a warm place for 30 minutes.

Spoon into non-stick muffin tins, filling them 2/3's full. Bake at 350° for 20 to 25 minutes. Makes 2 dozen muffins. Add 1/2 cup of raisins or other dried fruit for variety.

Brown Rice

1) Wash the rice by pouring cold water over 2 cups brown rice until any dust rises to the surface of the water. Pour off water, and repeat if necessary.

2) Add 4 cups of water to the clean rice and bring to a boil.

3) Cover saucepan and simmer slowly for 45 minutes or until all water is absorbed.

4) Turn off heat and let steam for 10 minutes.

5) Keep the rice in the refrigerator and reheat at mealtime. It can also be frozen and reheated.

Brownies

2 egg whites

1/2 cup honey
3/4 cup whole wheat flour
1/4 cup safflower or corn oil
1/4 cup cocoa mixed with 10 tablespoons
  lukewarm water
3/4 cup pecans, chopped
1 teaspoon vanilla

Beat egg whites until stiff. Mix honey, oil, cocoa (mixed with water) and vanilla together. Sift flour and stir into liquid ingredients. Add nuts. Fold egg whites into batter. Bake in a medium size, greased pan for 35 minutes in a preheated oven at 350°.

CHILI

1 lb tofu or ground turkey
4 cups fresh ripe tomatoes
2 cans red kidney beans with liquid
1 large onion, chopped
chili powder to taste
1 teaspoon ground cumin
1 clove of garlic, crushed

Sauté onion and garlic, then combine with the rest of the ingredients in a large heavy pot. Let simmer for 2 to 3 hours.

COD, BAKED

2 lb cod fish fillets or a
  whole codfish
paprika
sage
1/4 cup fish or chicken stock
1/3 cup white wine

Place cod in shallow, non-stick baking dish. Combine stock, wine, paprika and sage. Pour over cod and bake in a 350° oven until tender (between 8 to 10 minutes). Serve hot, garnished with chopped parsley.

COD AND RICE BAKE

1 lb chopped cod or other fish
3 stalks celery, sliced
1 onion, chopped
2 cups stewed tomatoes
1 cup uncooked brown rice, washed
1 1/2 cups low-salt mushroom soup

Preheat oven to 325°. Mix together above ingredients and bake for one hour and 20 minutes in a covered, non-stick casserole dish.

CORN PUDDING

2 cups corn
3 egg whites plus 1 egg yolk
1 cup skim milk
3 tablespoons whole wheat flour
dash cayenne pepper

Steam corn until tender. Drain and let cool. In a large bowl combine the corn with the skim milk. Beat the eggs and add to the mixture. Then add whole wheat flour and seasonings. Place in a lightly greased casserole dish. Put the dish in a shallow pan filled with hot water (about 1 inch of water is sufficient). Bake for 30 to 40 minutes at 400° or until a knife comes out clean.

COTTAGE CHEESE AND
CUCUMBER SALAD

2 cups low-fat cottage cheese
1 small cucumber
1 medium tomato, diced
2 green onions, finely chopped
4 lettuce leaves
freshly ground black pepper

paprika

Wash cucumber well and dice. Do not peel. Mix together cottage cheese, diced cucumber, tomato and green onion. Add pepper to taste. Serve on a lettuce leaf and sprinkle with paprika. Serves 4.

GRANOLA CRUNCH

4 cups rolled oats
3/4 cup chopped almonds
  or walnuts
1/2 cup wheat germ
1/2 cup powdered milk
1/4 cup safflower oil
1/4 cup honey
1 tablespoon vanilla
2/3 cup raisins or other dried fruit

Mix together all dry ingredients except the raisins. Combine and stir wet ingredients and add to dry mixture. Stir until evenly coated. Spread on baking sheet and cook for 25 minutes at 275°. Stir every 5 minutes. Remove and add raisins. Makes 20 servings.

GOURMET GREEN SALAD

4 large lettuce leaves
2 small yellow squash
1 stalk broccoli
1/2 cup bean sprouts
1/2 cup chick peas (garbanzo beans)
1/2 cup fresh mushrooms
1 medium tomato
1/2 cup fresh parsley

Tear lettuce into small pieces. Dice squash, broccoli, tomato and mushrooms into small pieces. Toss all ingredients together. Marinate in vinegar, olive oil and spice dressing.

HADDOCK, BAKED

2 lbs haddock fillets cut into 4-inch strips
paprika
1/4 teaspoon basil
1/8 teaspoon freshly ground black pepper
juice of 2 lemons

Pre-heat oven to 350°. Place fish in lightly greased baking dish with the other ingredients. Cover and bake for 15 minutes or until fish flakes easily.

KIDNEY BEAN SALAD

1 lb cooked kidney beans, drained
1 medium Spanish onion, diced
1/2 medium bell pepper, diced
2 tender celery stalks, diced
1/4 cup seasoned vinegar
1 tablespoon olive oil

Combine all ingredients and chill. This salad tastes best if left overnight in the refrigerater to maniate.

MACARONI AND CHEESE

1/2 lb macaroni (whole wheat is best)
1 cup low-fat ricotta cheese
1/8 teaspoon cayenne pepper
1/2 cup soft bread crumbs mixed with
 2 teaspoons low-fat margarine

Cook macaroni according to directions on package. Drain and rinse in cold water. Layer macaroni and cheese beginning with macaroni and ending with cheese. Pepper first layer of macaroni. Sprinkle bread crumbs over top of casserole dish. Bake at 350°

until top is browned.

MEAT LOAF

2 lbs lean ground beef
1 cup soft bread crumbs
1/4 cup unprocessed bran
1 1/4 cups skim milk
1 stalk celery, finely chopped
2 egg whites, beaten
1/3 cup onion, chopped
1 pinch each of pepper, mustard
  powder, sage
1 clove garlic, crushed

Sauté garlic, onion and celery then combine with the other ingredients. Shape into a loaf, place in loaf pan and top with 4 tablespoons tomato paste or low-salt tomato ketchup. Bake 1 1/2 hours at 350°.

OKRA SUPREME

2 lbs young, tender okra
4 large tomatoes, chopped
2 cloves garlic, crushed
1 teaspoon crushed oregano
freshly ground black pepper
juice of one lemon
1/4 to 1/2 cup salt-free tomato juice

Steam okra until tender. Place several tablespoons of water in a large frying pan. Pan fry garlic and onions in water over high heat. Add tomatoes, okra and tomato juice to onion and garlic mixture. Add seasonings, cover and simmer for 15 minutes. Cover with lemon juice. Serve hot.

Peppers Stuffed With Corn

6 medium bell peppers
3 cups corn
1 cup fresh tomato, diced
1 very small onion, diced
1/4 teaspoon freshly ground black pepper
1 clove garlic, crushed
1 teaspoon chili powder
3 tablespoons whole wheat flour
1 tablespoon vinegar

Remove tops from green peppers, then remove seeds and inside membrane. Parboil in covered saucepan for 5 minutes with vinegar added to the water. Combine remaining ingredients and spoon mixture into green peppers. Place in baking dish and bake at 375° for 35 minutes or until done.

Ratatouille

1 eggplant
3 zucchini
1 large onion
2 large tomatoes
1 clove garlic, crushed
1/2 teaspoon basil
2 tablespoons olive oil
whole wheat bread crumbs

Peel eggplant if skin is tough; otherwise wash and cut into 1/2 inch slices. Slice zucchini, onion and tomatoes. Layer eggplant, onion, zucchini and tomatoes. Mix seasonings with olive oil and pour over the casserole. Bake covered for 30 to 40 minutes at 350° or until vegetables are tender. Put whole wheat bread crumbs on top and brown.

RICE PUDDING

2 cups uncooked brown rice
4 cups skim milk
1/2 cup honey
2 teaspoons vanilla
2 egg whites
1/4 teaspoon cream of tartar
1/4 teaspoon nutmeg

Cook unsalted brown rice according to previous directions, but do not allow to steam at the end. Beat egg whites and cream of tartar until fluffy. Mix slightly undercooked brown rice, beaten egg whites, milk, honey, vanilla and nutmeg together. Bake in a non-stick pan or casserole dish at 350° for 1 hour. Makes 10 servings.

SALMON, STUFFED

4 salmon fillets
paprika
1 1/2 cups soft, whole wheat bread crumbs
1/4 cup celery, chopped
1 teaspoon grated onion
1 teaspoon chopped parsley
1 teaspoon tarragon
2 teaspoons of olive oil
juice of 1 lemon
1 lemon, sliced

Cut the fillets lengthwise in two pieces and lightly sprinkle with paprika. Combine bread crumbs, celery, onion, parsley and tarragon with the olive oil. Spread mixture on fish fillets and roll them up. Secure the rolls in place with toothpicks and brush with lemon juice. Place in a 375° oven for 30 minutes. Serve hot with lemon slices.

SLAW

4 cups shredded raw cabbage
1 tablespoon olive oil
1 teaspoon grated onion
2 tablespoons seasoned vinegar,
  or to taste

Mix cabbage and oil until cabbage is coated with oil. Add onion and toss to combine thoroughly. Add seasoned vinegar and mix. Best if left overnight in refrigerator before serving.

SPINACH SALAD

1 lb fresh spinach
2 1/2 tablespoons lemon juice
1/2 cup sliced mushrooms
  (preferably fresh)
1/2 cup grated raw carrots
1 1/2 tablespoons olive oil

Wash spinach thoroughly, removing all stems and drain off excess water. Combine remaining ingredients together in a cup. Pour mixture over the spinach salad, tossing thoroughly to coat. Serves 6.

SQUASH, STUFFED YELLOW

8 crookneck squash
2 egg whites, beaten
1 clove garlic, crushed
1 medium onion, chopped
2 tablespoons parsley, chopped
1 teaspoon ground basil
1/2 teaspoon ground savory
1 teaspoon olive oil

1 cup whole wheat bread crumbs

Saute garlic and onion in 2 tablespoons water until onion is clear. Trim squash, cut in half lengthwise and spoon out centers. Add squash centers and seasonings to non-stick frying pan and cook with olive oil until tender. Remove from heat. Add egg whites to squash mixture, spoon mixture into empty squash halves and sprinkle bread crumbs on top. Bake at 350° for 40 minutes or until tender. Serve hot.

THREE-BEAN SALAD

1 lb fresh green beans, cooked and drained
1 lb fresh wax beans, cooked and drained
1 lb dried kidney beans, cooked and drained
1 medium onion, sliced
1 small bell pepper, sliced
1/4 cup olive oil
1/2 teaspoon paprika

Combine beans, onion and bell pepper, set aside. Mix together remaing ingredients in a small bowl and mix well. Pour the seasoned oil over the bean mixture and toss well. Refrigerate overnight.

TOMATO RICE

1 1/2 cups brown rice, uncooked
2 cups water
1 1/4 cups unsalted tomato juice
3/4 cup celery, chopped

Bring water and tomato juice to a boil. Slowly add brown rice and celery. Cover and cook over low heat for 40 to 50 minutes, stirring occasionally. Remove cover during last 5 minutes of cooking.

TROUT, BAKED

2 lb trout fillets
juice of 2 lemons
1 lemon, sliced
paprika
1/8 teaspoon sage
chopped parsley

Place fillets in shallow baking pan. Brush with lemon juice and sprinkle with sage and paprika. Cook above the center of a 400° oven until fish flakes easily. Serve with lemon slices and parsley. Serves 4.

TUNA SALAD

4 small lettuce leaves
1 small can tuna, packed in water
2 hard cooked egg whites, chopped
1/2 small onion, grated
2 stalks celery, diced
1 teaspoon lemon juice

Drain tuna. Mix in celery and egg whites. Grate onion and add to mixture. Season with lemon juice. Serve on a lettuce leaf. Serves 4.

TUNA SALAD, TOSSED

1 medium head of lettuce
3 hard cooked egg whites, chopped
2 green onions, diced
1 medium tomato, finely diced
1 small can tuna, packed in water
2 tablespoons fine bran
freshly ground black pepper
paprika

Tear lettuce into small pieces. Drain tuna and toss with lettuce. Add remaining ingredients and toss well. Add pepper to taste. Sprinkle lightly with paprika.

VEGETABLE AND FRUIT TOSSED SALAD

1 bunch raw spinach
1/2 cup orange sections
2 green onions, finely chopped

Wash spinach thoroughly and tear into small pieces. Add remaining ingredients and toss well.

VEGETABLE DELIGHT

2 lbs fresh vegetables
2 egg whites
1/8 teaspoon freshly ground
  black pepper
2 tablespoons finely chopped parsley
2 tablespoons unprocessed bran

Pre-heat oven to 375°. Wash and trim vegetables as individually required. Mix bran with parsley and pepper. Dip vegetables in beaten egg whites and then in bran mixture. Place on non-stick cookie sheet and bake for 15 to 20 minutes or until brown. Serve hot.

VEGETABLE SALAD, MARINATED

1 cup fresh green beans (cooked and drained)
1/3 cup mushrooms (preferably fresh)
1 small head of cauliflower
1 small Spanish onion, thinly sliced
2 small carrots, sliced
4 stalks celery, diced
5 tablespoons vinegar
5 tablespoons olive oil
1/2 teaspoon freshly ground black pepper

Combine all ingredients. Toss well. Let stand 24 hours in the refrigerator. Mix occasionally. Serve cold.

aneurysm — An abnormal weakness in the wall of a blood vessel, usually an artery, that leads to ballooning. It is most often found in the aorta, which is the biggest artery in the body going from the heart through the chest and abdomen. An aneurysm can swell, enlarge, and eventually rupture.

angina pectoris — A sudden pain or pressure in the chest behind the breastbone which may radiate down the shoulder, neck, arm, hand or back, usually or mainly on the left side of the body. People with angina pectoris may also feel its sensations as burning, choking or indigestion. It is associated with insufficient blood flowing through narrowed coronary arteries which supply the heart muscle.

angioplasty — A technique used to widen narrowed arteries using a balloon catheter.

angiotensin — A hormone in the blood that raises blood pressure.

arteriosclerosis — Artery disease characterized by a loss of artery elasticity, deposits in the arteries, and hardening of the walls of the arteries leading to a decreased blood flow.

artery—Any blood vessel that carries blood away from the heart to the various organs and tissues of the body.

atheromas—Small raised plaques of mushy cholesterol, fat and foam cells on the inner walls of the arteries.

atherosclerosis—The deposit of cholesterol and other fatty, waxy substances on the inner walls of the arteries, often leading to narrowing and "hardening" of the arteries as scar tissue and calcification form.

blood pressure—The force exerted on the walls of arteries, veins and capillaries as the heart pumps blood through the body.

capillaries—Minute blood vessels that connect the smallest arteries to the smallest veins.

cardiac—Of or relating to the heart.

cardiac arrest—A heart attack or when productive heart beating stops.

cardiovascular—Pertaining to the heart and arteries.

cholesterol—A waxy fat present in some foods of animal origin; it is also manufacturered by the human body. Some cholesterol is needed by the body, but excessive amounts are associated with artery disease.

congestive heart failure — Occurs when the heart is unable to pump well enough to maintain good circulation. It often occurs because of a weakness in the heart muscle due to disease or a mechanical fault in the valves that control the flow of blood.

coronary heart disease or coronary artery disease — Narrowing or blockage of the coronary arteries which reduces the flow of blood to the heart muscle.

diastolic pressure — The pressure which remains in the blood vessels as the heart relaxes to allow for the flow of blood into its pumping chambers. The second number in a blood pressure reading.

diuretic — A drug that increases the flow of urine, more commonly known as a water pill.

drug interaction — One drug or other substance increasing, decreasing or changing the effects of another drug.

edema — Accumulation of fluid in the body.

ECG — See electrocardiogram.

electrocardiogram — A recording of the heart's electrical activity. By placing electrodes, usually with gel, on a person's arms, legs and chest, the heart's electrical activity can be monitored and recorded onto a strip of graph paper.

fiber — Dietary fiber, often called roughage, is the part of food that cannot be absorbed by the body. It is essential for proper elimination of body waste because it helps food move through the body. It is found in fruits, raw vegetables and whole grains. Highly processed foods, like white flour and sugar, contain little or no fiber.

generic name — The name given to the ingredient or ingredients in a drug as distinguished from brand names for drugs which may be trademarked by manufacturers.

heart attack — Heart failure or abnormal, weak functioning of the heart after its blood supply is abruptly cut off, usually due to narrowing of the arteries or a blood clot.

high blood pressure — See hypertension.

hypertension — Sustained high blood pressure of 140/90 or higher. The correct medical term for high blood pressure.

hypotension — Low blood pressure.

kidneys — Located at the back of the abdomen, kidneys are responsible for filtering the blood and removing the waste materials.

monounsaturated fats — Fatty acids that have one double or triple bond per molecule. They are easily split and other substances can join them. Found in olive oil, chicken, almonds and some other nuts.

nephrology — The study of the kidneys.

obesity — Being 20 to 40 percent heavier than your ideal weight.

oral contraceptive — A drug containing female hormones, usually synthetic estrogen and progesterone, to provide birth control by inhibiting the body's natural cycle of female hormone production which interferes with ovulation or the release of eggs.

polyunsaturated fats — Fatty acids that have more than one double or triple bond per molecule. Found in fish, soybean, safflower and corn oil. Polyunsaturated fats are usually soft or liquid at room temperature.

potassium — An essential mineral found in meat, potatoes, raisins, nuts, tomatoes, banana, milk and fruit. It serves as an electrolyte in the body and plays a part in the regulation of blood pressure.

renin — A substance released into the blood by the kidneys in response to stress that may change blood pressure.

salt — A common name for sodium chloride. It is used as a flavoring and a preservative. In the body, salt maintains fluid levels between the cells and the blood system and acts as an electrolyte to help chemical and electrical reactions.

saturated fat — A type of fat that raises blood cholesterol and trigylceride levels. All the atoms are joined by single bonds. Found in animal and dairy products such as beef, pork, lamb, veal, egg yolks, milk, butter, cheese, cream and a few vegetable fats, including coconut oil and hydrogenated vegetable shortening. Saturated fats are generally hard or solid at room temperature.

sphygmomanometer — An arm pressure cuff used to determine blood pressure.

stroke — An interruption of blood flow to an area of the brain, leading to damage and loss of function controlled by that area of the brain. Strokes can be caused by a blockage of a blood vessel in the brain or by bleeding from a blood vessel or an aneurysm into the brain. High blood pressure and smoking are the leading risk factors for stroke.

systolic pressure — The pressure which is produced as the heart contracts to pump blood out into the body. The first number in a blood pressure reading.

triglycerides — A type of fat carried throughout the body by the bloodstream. It is a particular combination of the three fatty acids. High-trigylceride levels are associated with overeating, obesity, high-fat or high-sugar diets, diabetes and coronary artery disease. High levels might be dangerous.

uremia — The build up of waste products in the blood, often associated with the progressive narrowing of the kidney blood vessels.

vein — Any blood vessel that carries blood back to the heart from various parts of the body.

vitamin — Organic chemical which is essential for normal chemical reactions in the body.

vitamin supplement — Extra vitamins used to supplement or add to those found in the diet.

water pill — see diuretic.